ISSUES IN
GRADUATE NURSING EDUCATION

Sylvia E. Hart, Editor

WY
18.5
I865
1987

►13749

Pub. No. 18-2196

nln

National League for Nursing • New York

ISBN 0-88737-381-X

Manufactured in the United States of America

CONTENTS

CONTRIBUTORS

Patricia R. Forni, PhD, RN, FAAN is dean, School of Nursing, Southern Illinois University at Edwardsville.

Sylvia E. Hart, PhD, RN is professor and dean, the University of Tennessee, Knoxville.

Frieda Holt, EdD, RN is professor and associate dean for graduate studies, University of Maryland, School of Nursing, Baltimore.

Mary Lou Jolly, EdD, RN is associate professor, The University of Tennessee, Knoxville.

Peri Rosenfeld, PhD is director, Division of Research, National League for Nursing, New York, New York.

Theresa Sharp, EdD, RN is associate professor, The University of Tennessee, Knoxville.

Jeanette Spero, PhD, RN, FAPHA is dean, College of Nursing and Health, University of Cincinnati, Ohio.

Patricia L. Starck, DSN, RN is professor and dean, School of Nursing, The University of Texas Health Science Center—Houston.

Marylou Yam, MA, MEd, RN is instructor, Felician College, Lodi, New Jersey.

1 INTRODUCTION

Sylvia E. Hart, PhD, RN

While the unresolved issues surrounding titling and licensue continue to preoccupy the nursing profession and others associated with the health care delivery system, it is appropriate and timely to examine the status and direction of graduate nursing education. Whatever the final decisions are relative to educational requirements for entry into professional nursing practice, it is clear that nursing's leadership will be provided by those who possess advanced knowledge in the discipline of nursing.

The number of master's degree programs in nursing has nearly doubled in the past ten years and will almost certainly surpass 200 by 1990. The growth in the number of doctoral programs in nursing has been even more dramatic. In 1975 there were ten doctoral programs in the United States. As this publication goes to press the number of such programs is approaching 50. And, while enrollments in undergraduate nursing programs are declining in a rather alarming manner, enrollments in graduate nursing programs continue to increase. Nearly 2,000 students are now enrolled in doctoral degree programs in nursing and almost 20,000 are enrolled in master's degree programs.

Since graduate nursing education is a relative newcomer on college and university campuses and because graduate program growth in nursing has been so prolific it is not surprising that there are wide variations in the structure, length, content, and emphasis of these programs as well as in degree requirements, degree designations, and accreditation status.

The contributors to this volume have examined the state of the art of graduate nursing education. In that process, they have brought focus and perspective to several key issues with which nurse educators, nurse administrators, and practicing nurses are grappling. How much research expertise should we develop in master's and doctorally prepared nurses? What is the appropriate length of and content for master's level nursing programs?

How good is the match between how nurses are prepared at the master's level and what they are employed to do? What are the essential distinctions between and among the various doctoral program models (N.D., Ed.D., D.N.S., D.N.Sc., Ph.D.)? Can these various models all be articulated into an understandable and marketable system for nursing education and practice? What role does or should NLN's accreditation program serve in the development of high quality, innovative nursing education programs at the graduate level? What is the current and emerging focus of doctoral dissertation research in nursing programs offered at that level?

These and other questions and issues are addressed in this publication and the challenges inherent in them are clear and compelling. But, while some of these issues are complex and multifaceted, it is encouraging, refreshing, and noteworthy that it is graduate nursing education that we are discussing, describing, and analyzing. That we have enough comparative data, enough collective experience and expertise, and enough confidence to identify, analyze, and address the questions, issues, and problems inherent in graduate nursing education is indeed a statement about the continuing emergence of nursing as an academic discipline and about nursing's rightful place in the mainstream of our academic communities. The final chapter which presents a review of recent doctoral dissertation titles authored by nurses lends further credence and legitimacy to nursing's expanding theoretical foundations that undergird nursing practice. There is no doubt that graduate education in nursing has had a tremendous impact on the profession. As more nurses with graduate preparation enter and remain in the nursing and health care work force the health care needs of society will be more fully met and the continuing positive development of the profession will be ensured.

2 THE MASTER'S-PREPARED NURSE IN THE MARKETPLACE: WHAT DO MASTER'S-PREPARED NURSES DO? WHAT SHOULD THEY DO?

Patricia L. Starck, RN, DSN

What do master's-prepared nurses do? They are the jack-of-all-trades. And this is not by accident, it is by design. One can readily understand this phenomenon considering the types and diversities of programs in master's-level nursing education. This chapter will describe the current state of diversity in master's preparation for nursing and discuss ambiguities in the roles of administration, clinical nurse specialization, nursing education, and nurse practitioners. A discussion of the different and complementary roles of physicians and nurses is given in order to clarify the services they offer and the research potential in their disciplines. The chapter will conclude with a description of present and future characteristics of master's education in nursing.

DIVERSITY AD INFINITUM

There is diversity in master's degree titles as well as in the content of curricula. Forni (1971) found 11 different degree titles from a survey of National League for Nursing (NLN)-accredited master's programs in 1984. These included MS, MSN (the two most common), MN, MA, MPH and MS, MA or MEd, MS or BS/MS, MSN and MS, MSN or MN, MNSc, MN, and MS.

In 1983, Williamson conducted an analysis of master's programs and found an "endless array of descriptions" (p. 99). Of the 109 graduate programs listed in the 1982–83 NLN publication, *Master's Education in Nursing,* there was very little standardization. There were more than 130 combinations of available areas of study, not including functional components. Williamson stated that the ambiguity and inconsistency in terminology is symptomatic of the lack of consensus regarding the structure of the discipline of nursing. She called for an effort to establish a cohesive classification and subclassification and recommended a forum to structure a national education plan for graduate education in nursing. The outcome would still allow for creativity and innovation but provide consistency of purpose and clear communication among nurses and with the broader community. A similar analysis done by this author in 1987 revealed that the situation has not improved; in fact, it has gotten even more complicated.

According to the latest directory of graduate nursing programs (National League for Nursing, 1986), there are 143 programs. There has been an addition of 130 program titles since Williamson's study in 1983, thus doubling the variety of titles, for a grand total of 257. The data in Table 1 reflect Williamson's original groupings (Groups 1–14). Group 15 lists new titles since Williamson's calculations. The numbers beside the title indicate the numbers of programs with that title. There are many one-of-a-kind titles. For example, there are 20 different titles to describe programs related to children (see Table 2). The question is, is each of the 20 programs substantially different; that is, are there at least 20 different types of products (graduates) needed to meet the needs of society, or are the differences merely semantic? Are they only slight variations, wherein all 20 programs have a common core? At any rate, it must be confusing to the public—the consumers.

TABLE 1.   Titles of Specific Areas of Study in Nursing (Groups 1-14, Williamson's Classification 1982-85; Group 15, additional titles, 1986-87)

GROUP 1
Maternal-Child 19
Maternal-Infant 6
Maternal-Infant Nurse Clinician 1
Maternal-Newborn 5
Maternal-Ob/Gyn Practitioner 1
Maternity 1
Maternity Clinical Nurse Specialist 2
Women/Infant Nursing 1

GROUP 2
Advanced Adult Nursing 1
Adult Acute Care Nurse Specialist 1
Adult Health 11
Adult Health and Illness 3
Adult Medicine

Adult Nurse Practitioner 6
Adult Nursing 18
Adult Nursing (Critical Care) 4
Medical-Surgical 52
Medical-Surgical Clinical Nurse Specialist 1
Medical-Surgical Nurse Clinician
Medical-Surgical/Psychiatric
Nursing of Adults with Biodissonance 2
Primary Care-Adults 3
Young and Middle Age Adults 2

GROUP 3
Adolescent Health 1
Advanced Child Health
Ambulatory Child Health Care

Table 1 continued.

(PNP) 7
Ambulatory Pediatrics
Child Health 7
Child Health Maintenance
Nursing Care of Children at Risk 2
Nursing Care-Children and
    Adolescents 1
Nursing of Children 12
Pediatrics 7
Pediatric Clinical Nurse Specialist 1
Primary Care-Pediatrics 2

GROUP 4
Ambulatory Women's Health
    Nurse Practitioner
Health Care of Women 1
Women's Health 6
Women's Health Care Track

GROUP 5
Community Health 58
Community Health Care Systems 4
Community Health-Family Nurse
    Practitioner or Clinical Specialist
Public Health (Community
    Health) 5

GROUP 6
Community Mental Health 9
Community Mental Health/
    Psychiatric 4
Gerontological Mental Health 2
Mental Health 9
Mental Health-Child
Mental Health Clinical Nurse
    Specialist
Mental Health Nurse Clinician
Psychiatric 9
Psychiatric/Adult-Child Clinical
    Specialist
Psychiatric/Mental Health 49
Psychiatric/Mental Health-Child/

Adolescent
Psychiatric/Mental Health Nurse
    Practitioner 1
Psychiatric Nurse Therapist
    (Clinician)
Psychiatry-Adult 1
Psychiatry-Child 1

GROUP 7
Advanced Family Nursing
Childbearing/Childrearing Family 2
Primary Care Family Nurse
    Clinician 1
Family Clinical Specialist 1
Family-Community Nursing 1
Family Health-Nurse Clinician
Family Nurse Practitioner 18
Family Nurse Specialist with
    Practitioner Skills 1
Family Nursing 3
Family Nursing in Urban
    Communities 1
Family-Primary Care

GROUP 8
Adult-Child Health 3
Child Health/Family Nurse
    Practitioner
Family Centered Child Nursing
Family Child Nursing
Parent-Child 28
Parent-Child Acute Care Nurse
    Specialist
Parent-Child Health 5

GROUP 9
Chronic Illness and Gerontology
Geriatric-Gerontology 6
Geriatric Nurse Practioner 9
Geriatric Nurse Practitioner and
    Clinical Specialist 2
Gerontological 22

Table 1 continued.

Gerontological Nurse Clinician 2
Gerontological Nursing Track
Gerontology 12
Nursing Care of Aged
Older Adult 1

GROUP 10
Occupational Health 5
Occupational Health Nurse Practitioner 3
School Health Nursing
School Nurse Clinician

GROUP 11
Acute Care 2
Critical Care 11
Critical Care Clinical Specialist 1
Long Term Care 1
Primary Ambulatory Care
Primary Care Clinician
Primary Care in Correctional
   Institutions
Primary Health Care 3
Primary Nursing Care in Society 1
Secondary Care 1
Secondary and Tertiary Care

GROUP 12
International Health
Transcultural Health

GROUP 13
Anesthesia 3
Anesthesia Nurse Practitioner 1
Burn and Trauma
Cancer 1
Cardiovascular 7
Developmental Disabilities 2
Diabetes Nursing 1
Emergency Care 1
Metabolic Problems
Neonatal/Perinatal 1

Oncology 17
Oncology Nurse Specialist
Pediatric Respiratory
Perinatal 3
Perinatal Nurse Practitioner
Perinatal Nurse Specialist 1
Physiological Nursing 2
Rehabilitation 2
Renal Problems
Respiratory Nursing
Spinal Cord Injury Nurse
   Practitioner

GROUP 14
Advanced Nursing Practice
Clinical Nursing 1
Health Nursing

**GROUP 15: ADDITIONAL
AREAS OF STUDY IN
1986–1987**
**Master's Education in Nursing:
Route to Opportunities in
Contemporary Nursing**
Acute Care Adult/Child 1
Acute Care Pediatric 1
Acute/Critical Care 1
Administration of Educational
   Programs 1
Administration of Nursing
   Services 9
Adolescent Health Care Clinical
   Specialist 1
Adult Acute 1
Adult Acute Care 1
Adult and Elderly 1
Adult Health Care 1
Adult Health Clinical Specialist 1
Adult Health Nursing 11
Adult Health Promotion and
   Illness Management 1
Adult Nursing (Medical) 1

Table 1 continued.

Adult Nursing (Surgical) 1
Adult Oncology 1
Adult Psychiatric/Mental Health 2
Adult/Elderly/Psychiatric/Mental
  Health 1
Advanced Medical/Surgical 1
Advanced Nursing Practicum 3
Aged 1
Ambulatory Care 1
Burn/Emergency/Trauma 1
Cardiopulmonary 1
Care of Women 1
Child 1
Child/Adolescent Clinical Nurse
  Specialist 1
Child/Adolescent/Psychiatric/
  Mental Health Specialist 1
Childbearing Family 1
Children/Adolescents 2
Chronic Disabilities 1
Chronically Mentally Ill 1
Clinical Practice 1
Clinical Specialist 22
Clinical Specialist in Primary Care
  Pediatrics 1
Clinical Specialist in Women's
  Primary Care 1
Community Health Home Health
  Care Delivery Systems 1
Community Health Nurse
  Practitioner 1
Community Health Nurse
  Specialist 2
Community/Family Health 1
Correctional Health 1
Cross-Cultural 1
Delivery of Nursing Services 1
Developmental Pediatric 1
Family Abuse 1
Family Health 3
Family Health Clinical Nurse
  Specialist 1

Family Mental Health 1
Family Nurse Clinician 4
Family Nursing 1
Family/Child 3
Family/Community Health 2
Gerontologic Primary Care 1
Gerontology Mental Health 21
Geropsychiatric 1
High-Risk Maternity 1
Home Health 1
Infection Control 1
International and Cross-Cultural
  Nursing 1
Late Adult 1
Management Administration 3
Maternal 1
Maternal Fetal Clinical Specialist 1
Maternal/Fetal 1
Maternal/Parent/Child 2
MBA/MSN 1
Mental Health Psychiatric 6
Middle Management 1
MSN with Latin American Studies 1
Neonatal 2
Neonatal Intensive Care Nursing 2
Neonatal Nurse Practitioner 1
Neuroscience Nursing 1
Nurse Practitioner 9
Nurse Specialist 1
Nurse-Midwifery 12
Nursing Administration 40
Nursing Care 1
Nursing Care of Adults 1
Nursing Care of Adults with
  Cancer 3
Nursing Care of Women 1
Nursing Care Systems
  Management 1
Nursing Education 9
Nursing Education Systems 1
Nursing for the Community 1
Nursing for the Family 1

Table 1 continued.

Nursing for the Individual 1
Nursing Health Policy 1
Nursing Management 3
Nursing of Adults 3
Nursing of Adults in Psychiatric/
  Mental Health Areas 1
Nursing of Adults with Physiologic
  Alterations 3
Nursing of Aging Adults
Nursing Science 1
Nursing Services Administration 10
Nursing, Parenting, and Families 1
Obstetric/Gynecologic Primary
  Care 1
Occupational Health Nurse
  Clinician 1
Parent-Child Health Clinical
  Specialist 1
Parent/Newborn 2
Patient Care Management 2
Pediatric Acute Care Clinical
  Specialist 1
Pediatric Oncology 3
Pediatric Pulmonary 1
Perinatal Clinical Specialist 1
Perinatal/Women's Health 1
Primary Ambulatory Nurse
  Practitioner 1
Primary Care 13
Primary Care in Women's Health 1
Primary Care of Adults 3
Primary Care of Children 3
Primary Health Nursing 1
Professorial in Nursing Education 1
Psychiatric/Community Mental
  Health 4
Psychiatric/Mental Health Clinical
  Specialist 1
Psychosocial 2
Psychosocial/Psychiatric Nurse
  Clinician 1
Public Policy Planner 1

Pulmonary 1
Research 1
Rural Community Health 1
School Nurse Practitioner 1
Severely Disturbed and Chronically
  Mentally Ill 1
Surgical 1
Teaching 4
Teaching of Nursing 6
The Adult and the Aging Family 1
The Growing Family 1
Trauma 1
Trauma/Critical Care 1

TABLE 2. Titles of Curricula Offered in the Area of Children, NLN-Accredited Schools (1986–87).

Child Health	Primary Care of Children
Advanced Child Health	Primary Care - Pediatric Nurse
Adolescent Health	Practitioner
Child and Adolescent Clinical	Pediatric Pulmonary
Nurse Specialist	Pediatric Oncology
Child and Adolescent Health	Developmental Pediatric Nursing
Nursing of Children	Acute Care Pediatrics
Nursing Care of Children	Pediatric Primary Care
Nusing of Children and Adolescents	School Nurse Practitioner
Nursing of Children at Risk	Advanced Nursing Practice -
Advanced Nursing Practice - Child	Children and Adolescents
	Nurse Educator - Parent - Child

Likewise, consider the diversity in titles of curricula offered in the area of nursing administration. There are 21 variations in title (NLN, 1986), see Table 3. Is the corporate headhunter, who is presented with this array of degrees, able to discern differences or determine which graduates are best prepared? Or does the variety suggest there is no standardization of the product? An MBA communicates a standard image, but an MSN does not. Is this nurse education plethora, pluralism in the extreme? Can any other discipline boast such creative productivity on the part of educators?

TABLE 3. Titles of Curricula Offered in Nursing Administration, NLN-Accredited Schools (1986–87).

Nursing Administration	Nursing Administration/
Nursing Service Administration	Supervision
Nursing Services Administration	Administration in Nursing
Nursing Systems Administration	Manager
Administration of Nursing Services	Management Administration
Nursing Administrators	Patient Care Management
Service Administration	Management of Nursing in Health
Administration of Nursing	Agencies
Administration of Nursing Services	Nursing Management
Administration of Nursing Health	Delivery of Nursing Services
Services	Leadership in Nursing Practice
	MBA/MSN
	Home Health Care Delivery Systems

Source of Diversity

From what source do all these hybrids emerge? Is it from marketplace feasibility studies based on needs and demands? Common sense would lead one to believe not, or else the marketplace differs widely according to geographic location. Although a feasibility study that demonstrates need and demand usually accompanies requests for new programs, rarely does it help refine curricular decisions. No, the type of curricular focus a master's program has is usually based on at least two factors: (1) the philosophy of the school and parent institution and (2) the resources available, including faculty expertise.

Types of Curricular Diversity

In general, master's programs follow one of three routes: (1) a clinical focus, (2) a role preparation focus, or (3) an integrated focus. Examples of each, respectively, are (1) oncology nursing, (2) nursing administration, or (3) transcultural nursing. Programs often combine these components so that a student has both a clinical focus and a role preparation concentration. To further complicate matters, some programs offer a major in transcultural nursing, while others claim to integrate transcultural nursing throughout the curriculum regardless of the clinical focus. Moreover, another mind-boggling design is to have a role preparation choice as the major without a specialized clinical focus. That is, one's degree may be in nursing administration without advanced clinical knowledge at a specialized level. To further complicate matters, new types of programs are springing up every year. These new programs reflect certain current health problems, for example, correctional health care. Then there are those for specific populations, such as women's health care.

The same type of bizarre diversity is reflected in organizational structures of schools of nursing. No two are alike. What some schools call departments of adult health, other may call physiological or psychosocial nursing, and still others call medical-surgical nursing. Does the diversity represent creativity and academic freedom? Perhaps to a degree, but my opinion is that our lack of anything that remotely resembles uniformity is reflective of the state-of-the-art of our body of knowledge; that is, specific domains to form parts of the whole. Is there any other well-established discipline that has a pattern remotely like the diversity of nursing graduate education?

Whereas diversity in clinical specialization may be linked to local clinical resources, one might expect more uniformity in role preparation. However, that is not the case. Diversity in nursing administration and the roles of clinical nurse specialist, nurse educator, and nurse practitioner will be discussed.

Diversity Within Nursing Administration Programs

The diversity in nursing administration is reflected in preparation and curricular content. This section will describe these differences as well as advocate an ideal model and describe nurse administrator effectiveness.

The dilemma of nurse administrator preparation. There is no disagreement that the health care world of today needs well-prepared nurses with expertise in administration/management. The disagreement is on how this preparation should take place. There are at least four models found in today's educational system.

1. **The registered nurse with a baccalaureate degree in nursing or in a non-nursing field obtains a non-nursing master's degree in an administration discipline, such as a master's in business administration, or a master's in health care administration.**

   This model is decried by nursing educators; however, many nurses in practice hold such degrees as status symbols. Indeed, many were advised by fellow professionals to deliberately seek a non-nursing master's degree for more credibility among the larger world of managers. The latest argument for a non-nursing master's degree is that it will be more beneficial in assisting the nurse to move up the corporate health care ladder, where administrative responsibilities may extend beyond nursing to other clinical services, such as pharmacy, physical therapy, and so forth.

2. **A master's degree in nursing with a clinical specialty as well as role preparation in administration.**

   This degree includes a selected area of specialization in a clinical field, such as critical care nursing, as well as a sequence of courses in nursing administration. Type of content and distribution of credit vary widely by school; however, a prototype might be the majority of courses focusing on the clinical specialty, with a minor in nursing administration. The curriculum would typically also include a set of courses in theory, research, and cognates, such as pathophysiology. This pattern clearly intends to prepare a clinical administrator; one with expert power in the clinical specialty. Time in the curriculum for administrator preparation is, of necessity, limited.

3. **A master's in nursing degree with a specialty in nursing administration.**

   Perhaps the model representing the most controversy among nursing educators is this curriculum focused solely on role preparation and devoid of any specific clinical area of expertise. Believers in this model base its structure on the philosophy that nursing administration is, in and of itself, a specialized area of knowledge. The graduates of this program are quickly assimilated into the work world. Their expertise in nursing administration would be expected to be greater than those with a model 2 type of degree since almost all the curriculum has been focused in this area. However, this administrator may lack expert power when dealing with highly specialized clinical areas.

4. A joint or dual degree of nursing and administration.

A master's degree with a specialty in clinical nursing combined with a degree in a non-nursing administrative field describes this model. An example is the MSN/MBA, a very prestigious education with highly sought after graduates. However, barriers to this plan include longer time and increased costs to complete the degree. It is also reported that nurses have difficulty meeting prerequisites in the business school and admission scores on the GMAT.

The ideal model of nursing administration programs. Rather than debate the advantages and disadvantages of each model, it may be more helpful to start with the "ideal model" concept. What attributes would the ideal program have? That is, what would be the expected outcomes from a graduate of an ideal program? The following characteristics might be considered ideal:

- State-of-the-art knowledge level of administrative theory and organizational behaviors.

- Competencies in all areas of administration, including budgeting, personnel management, strategic planning, and so forth.

- Abilities to communicate and interact up and down the organizational structure and within various disciplines.

- Skills in collaboration and negotiation.

- Resource acquisition (including fundraising) and management.

- Vision and creativity.

- Ethical behaviors, demonstrating knowledge of legal implications.

- Ability to utilize constantly changing technology, such as computers, and so forth.

- A basic knowledge of generalist nursing care in all clinical areas.

- A broad knowledge in emerging nursing issues in all clinical specialties sufficient to communicate with specialized caregivers (but without depth in any one clinical specialty).

- Transcultural awareness of the client population served as well as needs of the caregivers.

The makings of nurse administrator effectiveness. In a study of the effectiveness of directors of nursing, Freund (1985) found that it was the equal combination of management and clinical nursing that resulted in success. However, neither the directors of nursing nor the chief executive officer stressed knowledge of advanced clinical practice, but rather general knowledge of clinical practice, the nursing profession, and the health care field. In this study, "effectiveness" was not defined, rather characteristics were elicited by the respondents. The results were divided into eight categories:

- Flexibility/negotiation/compromise.
- Total organization view.
- Human management skill.
- General management/health/nursing knowledge.
- Political savvy.
- CEO support.
- Medical staff relations.
- Other.

The author of the study made three recommendations for curricular inclusion:

1. Solid base in the field of management, including organizational theory and organizational behavior, accounting, finance, productivity, personnel administration and computer literacy, or:
    - Fiscal management.
    - Resource management.
    - Information management.
2. Organizational politics.
3. Content related to general knowledge of nursing practice, nursing profession, and the health industry.

The debate over curricular content. Cleland (1984) and colleagues at Wayne State University operate on the belief that management-related content belongs in each curricular level from baccalaureate to doctorate, with a specialist certificate program between master's and doctorate and have devised an articulated model. Curricular components are goals and evaluation, finance, human resources, management, nursing, and research.

Poulin (1984) likewise agrees that basic management should be introduced at the baccalaureate level, beginning level practice for nursing administration at the master's level, and advanced preparation at the doctoral level.

However, Poulin disagrees with the need for an administrator to be prepared at the advanced clinical level. "The issue of clinical competence continues to be debated. It is kept alive and well mainly by educators. This may be symptomatic of an anti-administration attitude. . . The issue of clinical competence must be put to rest. What is needed are programs that help students strengthen their self-concept as professional nurses and as representatives of nursing in agencies" (p. 39). And so the debate continues and remains unresolved. Some educators believe this disagreement is good; it gives students a choice. However, it also can give employers a headache when trying to establish a management team whose members come from different philosophical stances.

The dilemma is not unlike that in the field of education which for years has vacillated between teacher preparation in the area of content specialty (what to teach), in the area of education (how to teach), or some combination (A Nation Prepared, 1986). It is interesting to note that nursing has long since abandoned the master's in education as appropriate for teaching nursing. Today, we require faculty to have degrees in the area of content specialty. After all, you cannot teach what you do not know. The argument follows that neither can you manage clinical care that you do not understand. This author speaks in favor of advanced clinical knowledge in all programs preparing nursing administrators. Thus, the closest thing to the ideal model for this author is the dual degree, MSN/MBA.

Diversity in Clinical Nurse Specialists

Sparacino (1983) traced the history of the clinical nurse specialist (CNS) from the first master's program in 1954. Almost three decades later there is still ambiguity about how the product should be utilized, whether in a line position or a staff position (Walker, 1986); how much, if any, administrative responsibility (Harrell & McCullock, 1986); whether the position is cost-effective (Walker, 1986); and when the functions leave nursing and extend to physicians' responsibilities. Furthermore, "the diversity of the role seems limitless" (Robichaud & Hamric, 1986, p. 31). Nevertheless, the clinical nurse specialist is well respected for advanced clinical practice knowledge and skills in influencing the quality of care in specialty areas. Role components include patient care, consultation, education, administration, professional development, and research, as specified by Robichaud and Hamric (1986). These authors developed operational definitions for each of these role components as the basis for a time document evaluative instrument.

After a comprehensive review of the research and education literature, Sparacino (1983) concluded that there was still no consensus on the definition of the role of the CNS. Thus, research as to the professional accountability of the role and the scientific basis of nursing practice is inhibited.

Ambiguity of roles for clinical nurse specialists. Hall (1986) describes the CNS as a nurse with a master's degree and expertise in a special clinical area of nursing whose role developed "to help the educated, experienced nurse to keep in touch with the patient and patient-centered activities" (p. 175). In characterizing the role of the CNS in an emergency department where the CNS has developed nursing care standards, Hall stated that "the CNS spends time in direct care to serve as a role model for the staff" (p. 175). Harrell and McCulloch (1986) make a case for the CNS becoming a "role model to staff nurses for autonomous functioning by demonstrating collaboration between the physicians and staff nurse, gradually testing expanded roles" (p. 46). They further state that the "knowledge base of the CNS, coupled with freedom from daily patient care duties allow the CNS to examine new options for patient care and to take an objective look at patient care problems and staff problems" (p. 47).

Hoffman and Fonteyn (1986) advocate that CNSs "expand their customer base to survive hard economic times" and that they apply "basic marketing strategies [that] will enhance their job security" (p. 140). In this report, CNSs established themselves as consultants, charged fees for services ordered by physicians, documented their activities on a special chart sheet labeled "Patient Education," distributed business cards to patients and families, dressed in street clothes with a white lab coat and identifying name tag. However, when the CNS gave direct patient care "she wore a traditional white nursing uniform or scrub suit" (p. 143).

Thus, it would seem that the CNS usually gives patient care from afar, through others. In the event the CNS gives care directly, the primary purpose is not to take care of the patient but to demonstrate to others how good care should be given. This phenomenon, coupled with the fact that most doctorally prepared nurses are teaching or conducting research, gives nursing the unique distinction among clinical disciplines that the more education one gets, the farther away from the patient one gets.

Barriers for clinical nurse specialists. This confusion about the role of the CNS is further elucidated by Walker (1986) who pointed out that some nursing service administrators see the CNS as a threat to their professional competence, based on the misunderstanding that the CNS assumes management as well as clinical responsibilities. In addition to competition with nursing administrators, the CNS faces conflict and rivalry from staff nurses (Harrell & McCulloch, 1986). The CNSs role of evaluating care through quality assurance studies and clinical research projects places the CNS in the role of judge of staff nurses and the care they give. Thus, not only are the CNSs disenfranchised from the patient; they are also disenfranchised from the very target population they are designed to help—the nursing staff. Unlike nursing direct caregivers, they must market themselves to demonstrate their usefulness.

Diversity in Nurse Educator Programs

Programs that prepare nurses at the master's degree level for teaching usually do so as secondary to a clinical area (NLN, 1986). These roles may include patient teaching, in-service staff development teaching, continuing education for practicing nurses, and teaching in schools of nursing.

Diversity in types of programs (NLN, 1986) appears largely semantic—teaching nursing, teaching of nursing, nurse educator. However, the approach and content may vary widely across programs.

In baccalaureate and higher degree nursing programs, expectation for the teaching role is doctoral level preparation. Most programs advertising for faculty also emphasize a clinical specialty at the master's level. Thus, the function of the master's degree, once considered a terminal degree for nursing faculty, now appears largely to be an intermediate step.

Diversity in Nurse Practitioner Programs

Nurse practitioners (NPs), as providers of basic and/or specialized health services, are now licensed in every state (Sweet, 1986). Unlike the clinical nurse specialist, the role of the nurse practitioner to give direct patient care is clear and undisputed. Whereas the CNS usually works with groups of individuals (whether patient, family, or staff), the nurse practitioner works one-on-one with a patient, which may or may not include the family. Furthermore, the type of care is different, that is, nurse practitioners generally focus on primary care, whereas the CNS is more likely to focus on secondary or tertiary care. Settings are also different, as is the degree of autonomy created by the setting.

Ginzberg (1987) predicts a favorable future for nurse practitioners. He believes the public will increasingly find that NPs better meet some of their needs than physicians; however, physician surplus will no doubt result in increasing competition.

The types of curriculum offerings for nurse practitioners are diverse, ranging in titles from those that suggest generalist (family nurse practitioner) to specific (occupational health nurse practitioner). The diversity of programs among NLN-accredited schools in 1986 is shown in Table 4.

TABLE 4.   Titles of Curricula Offered in the Area of Nurse Practitioner, NLN-Accredited Schools (1986–87).

Family Nurse Practitioner
Primary Care Nurse Practitioner
Adult Nurse Practitioner
Primary Ambulatory Care Nurse Practitioner
Family Health Nurse Specialist with Nurse Practitioner Skills
Community Nurse Practitioner
School Nurse Practitioner
Nurse Practitioner, family
Health Nursing–Nurse Practitioner
Gerontology Nurse Practitioner

Geriatric Nurse Practitioner
Obstetrics–Gynecological Nurse Practitioner
Pediatric Nurse Practitioner
Psychiatric/Mental Health Nurse Practitioner
Occupational Health Nurse Practitioner
Anesthesia Nurse Practitioner
Neonatal Nurse Practitioner
Nurse Practitioner: Maternal and Women's Health

One of the greatest strengths of the NP is clinical assessment. Other skills include treatment of common health problems, preventive care, and chronic maintenance care. Health teaching is a component of all aspects of care.

A challenge facing nurse practitioners today is to document their cost effectiveness through sound research to prepare for the mounting struggle over legal authority to practice independently. These data must be in place as issues of competitiveness with other providers increase.

One of the issues that must be faced and clarified in graduate nursing education is that of nurse-physician relationships and territoriality. The next section discusses this issue from the perspectives of complementarity of roles as well as differences in practice as reflective in research questions for nurses and physicians.

NURSE-PHYSICIAN ROLES: IMPACT OF GRADUATE NURSING EDUCATION

Unfortunately, in the public's mind, the difference between physician and nurse is that the former knows more and can do more. In this conceptualization, the brighter a nurse is and the more experience he or she has, the more ''like'' a physician he or she becomes. To counteract this perception, it is necessary to clarify roles of the physician and of the nurse, and especially the nurse who is steeped in clinical science knowledge and is becoming increasingly skillful.

Complementary Roles

In a model that depicts roles of physician and nurse as complementary, there are the unique aspects of each role, as well as shared aspects. There are at least four areas where nurse-physician roles can be delineated. First, physicians focus on cure, nurses add caring. We are beginning to study phenomenon to determine whether or not caring can actually accelerate healing. Caring behaviors have been described by Krueter (1957) as tending to another, being with another, giving heed to another's responses, guarding another from danger, providing for another's needs and wants with compassion, tenderness, consideration, respect, and concern. Noncaring behaviors include being in a hurry, just doing a job, being rough to and belittling a patient, not responding, and treating patients as objects (Riemen, 1986). Second, whereas physicians concentrate on pathology, nurses add concerns for psychosocial aspects of the individual and/or group. New findings that a hardy personality disposition can buffer the effects of stress on the individual (Kobasa, Maddi, & Kahn, 1982; Pines, 1980; Wiebe & McCollum, 1986) are very significant for nursing care, which involves the psychosocial aspects of the care plan. The new field of psychoneuroimmunology is documenting scientific evidence that how people appraise stressful events and react to them affects their resistance to disease at a cellular level (Justice, 1987). The nurse's role in influencing attitudes and reactions to stress is unquestionable. Third, physicians traditionally focus on illness, whereas nurses add wellness and wholeness to care. And fourth, physicians have short-term, intermittent contact, while nurses, at least those in hospital and long-term care settings, add long-term, continuity of care. Thus, nurse-physician roles are complementary in at least four dimensions:

- care–cure
- psychosocial–pathological dimensions of care
- wellness–illness
- long-term care–short-term care

Nurse-Physician Practice: Differences in Research Questions

How then do these differences manifest themselves in practice roles of the physician and a graduate-prepared nurse? Nowhere is the contrast of physician and nurse more evident than in the research questions generated as a result of the thinking and schooling of these two professionals. To illustrate this point, a set of research questions from the perspectives of both the nurse and the physician in each of the four dimensions was developed and may be found in Table 5. It should be obvious that to achieve comprehensiveness, both perspectives must be incorporated into approaches to health problems. As we continue to struggle with upgrading the image of nursing, attention must be given to the differences in nursing practice and medical practice, differences that are parallel and equitable in importance of the outcome.

TABLE 5. Research Questions from Physician-Nurse Perspectives (AIDS).

PHYSICIANS	NURSES
CURE	CARE
What kind of virus carries this disease? How can we develop a vaccine?	What determines which people who harbor the virus succumb to AIDS? How does the hardiness factor work

in these cases?

What strategies of patient education about preventions are more likely to change behaviors? What are the problems and needs of patients and their support system when the patient is dying of AIDS?

ILLNESS

What are the genetic predispositions of people who succumb to this disease? What factors or etiological agents are involved? What are the signs and symptoms of this disease that aid diagnosis and what other diseases must be ruled out? What are the treatment options—medical and/or surgical?

WELLNESS

How can people optimize their chances for maintaining wellness— managing stress, life-style, habits, and so forth? What is normal and what are the parameters of normality? What do patients with chronic illness have to be taught to stay as healthy as possible? When a patient is healing (e.g., from surgery) what accelerates the process or presents complications? How can this person and family members who are predisposed to the same condition avoid the problems?

How can patients behaviorally augment their immune systems?

PATHOLOGICAL DIMENSIONS

What is the organism and how does it affect the host? How are the pathological changes manifest at the cell level? How do these changes affect the entire body systems? How can we fix the pathology?

PSYCHOSOCIAL DIMENSIONS

How is this individual reacting to the occurrences of pathology? What are the psychosocial ramifications of this change in the body? How can we bolster the patient's motivation, coping abilities, human spirit to control or affect getting well and staying well?

SHORT TERM

What do the history and physical exam suggest for diagnosis? What treatment is appropriate? What overt signs of improvement/deterioration can be seen? After the major problem has been fixed, what are the smaller problems or needs over the course of healing? What is the cost/benefit

LONG TERM

What are the subtle factors that impinge on this person's state of health? How is the patient responding to treatment? Based on experience, what would enhance and/or accelerate the healing process? What are the overt and covert signs that the fixing of the major problem is and ratio of available treatment for this individual (based on age, degree of pathology, and so forth)?

remains uncomplicated? How can the patient be assisted to maintain hope and use his/her strength to participate in the plan of care: How can the nurse assist the patient's family to understand the health problems and options available? How can plans be made for quality of care and cost effectiveness?

CONCLUSIONS

What then are the present characteristics of graduate education in nursing? As rapid changes take place in the health care system, what should future characteristics be?

Present Characteristics of Master's Nursing Education

The third revision of *Characteristics of Master's Education in Nursing,* adopted on June 16, 1987 at the National League for Nursing convention held in Washington, DC, emphasizes both advanced nursing practice and advanced role preparation, regardless of which one is the primary focus. The document advocates advanced practice preparation for both generalized and specialized areas of study. Role preparation encompasses clinical specialists, nurse practitioners, administrators, and educators. The blend of advanced clinical practice and role preparation should produce outcomes of leadership, management, teaching, research, intellectual curiosity, creative inquiry, collaborative and consultative skills, and professionalism. Graduates must be able to articulate the value of specialized nursing services as contrasted to or in combination with services of physicians and/or other providers.

A graduate-level curriculum that includes theory, research, cognates in other disciplines, clinical knowledge, and applications in role development will produce a graduate with the foundation for doctoral study and for continued professional development. It becomes even more important in the face of the variety of clinical specializations and role preparation to have a well-conceptualized curricular schema that provides a common core of learning experiences for all students and provides integrity and consistency of the curriculum. The schema is also essential for systematic program evaluation.

The faculty–student relationship in graduate programs is important to the learning process. A peer relationship develops which promotes collegiality with nurses as well as members of other disciplines.

Future Characteristics of Master's Nursing Education

The rapidly changing scene of the health care system will challenge nurses with graduate-level preparation. The prospective payment system is bringing about a trend towards managed care; that is, care that is planned and contracted for based on baseline needs. The field of home care, and often hospital-type care in the home, will require increasing knowledge level and clinical competency with greater independence and autonomy in making clinical judgments.

The increasing knowledge from psychoneuroimmunology offers an opportunity for nurses to document the effects of caring, attitude motivation, and inspiration of hope as related to patient outcome. The link between essential components of the nurse–patient relationship and self-healing or control of progress can be studied through carefully designed research projects. The master's-prepared caregiver is in an excellent position to assist in mobilizing these forces.

The American Nurses' Association in its publication *New Organizational Models and Financial Arrangements for Nursing Services* (LeBar & McKibben, 1986) offered new ideas for nursing service delivery. Six models were presented for managed care:

Model A. Nursing service company providing organized nursing services to institutions and agencies.

Model B. Organized nursing service as an affiliate of an existing hospital.

Model C. Community-based nursing center.

Model D. Nursing center directed toward a specific phenomenon.

Model E. Independent nursing practice.

Model F. Private case management service.

Implementation of these models will require nurses with clinical knowledge as well as business skills. Likewise, knowledge of legalities, accounting, and marketing will be necessary as will political skills in dealing with the inevitable resistance from other health care providers.

The future for master's-prepared nurses is bright, particularly at the level of direct patient care where skills are best utilized for cost effectiveness. The diversity in types of programs may have exceeded "overkill." Programs should be more standardized so the consumers can know what the product (the graduate) is capable of in terms of delivery of services. Distinguishing nursing roles and services from those physicians is timely, as public attention focuses on the importance of caring in accelerating healing. Innovative models of practice present challenging opportunities. Graduate preparation that is strong, solid, clear, and distinct is the way to achieve the professional mission of service to others.

REFERENCES

A nation prepared: Teachers for the 21st century. The Report of the Task Force on Teaching as a Profession. Carnegie Forum on Education and the Economy. May, 1986.

Characteristics of master's education in nursing, third revision. (1986). National League for Nursing Convention, Washington, DC: Adopted June 16, 1987.

Cleland, V. (1984). An articulated model for preparing nursing administrators. *Journal of Nursing Administration, 14* (10), 23–31.

Forni, P. (1987). Nursing's diverse master's programs: The state of the art. *Nursing and Health Care, 8* (2), 70–75.

Freund, C. M. (1985). Director of nursing effectiveness: DON and CEO perspectives and implications for education. *Journal of Nursing Administration, 15* (6), 25–30.

Ginzberg, E. (1987). New economic climate breeds new markets. *Nursing and Health Care, 8* (3), 139.

Hall, M. M. (1984). A clinical nurse specialist for your emergency department? *Journal of Emergency Nursing, 10* (3), 175–177.

Harrell, J., & McCullock, S. (1986). The role of the clinical nurse specialist: Problems and situations. *Journal of Nursing Administration, 16* (10), 44–48.

Hoffman, S. E., & Fonteyn, M. E. (1986). Marketing the clinical nurse specialist. *Nursing Economics, 4* (3), 140–144.

Justice, B. (1987). *Who gets sick: Thinking and health.* Houston: Peak Press.

Kobasa, S. C., Maddi, S. R., & Kahn, S. (1982). Hardiness and health: A prospective study. *Journal of Personality and Social Psychology, 42* (1), 168–177.

Kreuter, F. (1957). What is good nursing care? *Nursing Outlook, 5* (5), 302.

LaBar, C. & McKibbin, R. (1986). *New organizational models and financial arrangements for nursing services.* Kansas City, Missouri: American Nurses' Association.

National League for Nursing, Council of Baccalaureate and Higher Degree Programs. (1986). *Master's education in nursing: Route to opportunities in contemporary nursing, 1986–1987.* New York: Author.

Pines, M. (1980). Psychological hardiness: The role of challenge in health. *Psychology Today, 14* (12), 35–44, 98.

Poulin, M. S. (1984). Future directions for nursing administration. *Journal of Nursing Administration, 14* (3), 37–41.

Riemen, D. J. (1986). Noncaring and caring in the clinical setting: Patients' descriptions. *Topics in Clinical Nursing, 8* (2), 30–36.

Robichaud, A., & Hamric, A. B. (1986). Time documentation of clinical nurse specialist activities. *Journal of Nursing Administration, 16* (1), 31–36.

Sparacino, P (1986). The clinical nurse specialist. In W. L. Holzemer (Ed.), *Review of research in nursing education, Volume I* (pp. 65–88). New York: National League for Nursing.

Sweet, J. B. (1986).The cost effectiveness of nurse practitioners. *Nursing Economics, 4* (4), 190–193.

Walker, M. L. (1986). How nursing service administrators view clinical nurse specialists. *Nursing Management, 17* (3), 52–54.

Wiebe, D. J., & McCollum, D. M. (1986). Health practices and hardiness as mediators in the stress-illness relationship. *Health Psychology, 5* (5), 425–438.

Williamson, J. A. (1983). Master's education: A need for nomenclature. *Image: The Journal of Nursing Scholarship, XV* (4), 99–101.

3 MASTER'S-PREPARED NURSES: SOCIETAL NEEDS AND EDUCATIONAL REALITIES

Mary Lue Jolly, EdD, RN
Sylvia E. Hart, PhD, RN

The development of master's-level programs in nursing parallels several driving forces that include but are not limited to social, governmental, technological, economic, educational, professional, and deomographic influences. These forces not only led to the development of master's-level nursing programs, but also strongly influenced and helped shape master's program content, program focus, program requirements, and program options. A review of these driving forces and their influence on past, present, and future directions in nursing education at the master's level reveals a developmental history that is beginning to reflect a more realistic balance between what master's prepared nurses do and how they are educated.

THE NEED FOR MASTER'S PREPARED NURSES

Governmental Influences

The federal government is one major force that has influenced the need for master's-level nursing programs. For example, the Surgeon General's Report (United States Public Health Service, 1963), a comprehensive analysis of national, regional, and state needs for nurses, recommended that graduations from master's programs be tripled by 1970. In 1979, after 15 years of generous allocations of federal dollars to nursing programs, the Congress of the United States mandated a study of nursing and nursing education for a threefold purpose. One of the objectives was to obtain an evaluation of the need for the federal government to continue to provide funds for nursing education. The Institute of Medicine of the National Academy of Sciences, commissioned to conduct the study, published its findings in 1983 under the title *Nursing and Nursing Education: Public Policies and Private Actions.* This document, frequently referred to as "the IOM Study," contains 21 recommendations. One of the most important of these recommendations cited the critical need for nurses who are prepared at the master's level. The committee identified a wide range of problems that can be alleviated only by substantially increasing the number of master's prepared nurses for nursing practice and for nursing education. The authors of this report emphasized the importance of graduate education in nursing when they stated that "RNs with high quality graduate education are a scarce national resource and...their education merits continuing federal support" (p. 10). The report emphasized that the most crucial need for nursing today is greater numbers of qualified practitioners, managers, and educators who will move nursing toward the professional status it must achieve. Clearly, national mandates based on comprehensive studies of nursing (accompanied as they were with the allocation of federal dollars for graduate nursing education) greatly accelerated the production of master's prepared nurses.

Technological Influences

Another driving force that has contributed to the need for more nurses prepared at the master's level is the rapid expansion of scientific knowledge coupled with the development of sophisticated technology and its application to health care. One need only walk into an intensive care unit or even into a general hospital patient unit to be struck by the elaborate equipment and gadgetry that is apparent everywhere. It is now possible to monitor an individual's every bodily function with a remarkable degree of accuracy and, based on the data constantly being generated, to make predictions about the person's condition. The ability of physicians and health team members to transplant vital organs, insert artificial parts, and use complex medications to prevent or reverse inflammatory or infectious processes is becoming commonplace.

These scientific and technological developments have extended the average life expectancy of our total population and have significantly increased the complexity of hospital care for the acutely ill. The kind and level of nursing care now required in most hospitals is so advanced and comprehensive that much of it cannot be delegated to nurses who are not prepared at the graduate level.

The complexity of care of the aged in acute-care facilities is particularly significant. Not only is it estimated that life expectancy will continue to increase each year but it is also projected that by the year 2000, 50 percent of all health care costs will be related to the care and treatment of people age 65 or older (Spitzer & Davivier, 1987). Increased longevity coupled with a quality existence is indeed a positive outcome with significant economic

implications. The cost effective treatment and management modalities required are best provided by well-educated nurses who, by virtue of their advanced education and expertise, can bring creative and effective approaches to the delivery of cost-effective health and nursing services.

The impact of technology on longevity with the consequent need for nurses prepared at the master's level is further underlined by examining the status of the Medicare program. In 1965 when the Medicare program began under the Social Security system it was established to provide health care services for disabled individuals and/or those who reached age 65. The program has been stretched beyond its limits. The federal government now pays 60 to 70 percent of the total health care bill for the United States. It is not surprising, therefore, that those associated with federal health care policy have a high level of interest in reducing the cost of health care. One result of that interest has been a shift from a retrospective payment system to the much more controlled and specific prospective payment known as diagnostic related groups (DRGs). This approach, which offers incentives to shorten the hospital stay of patients, also has significant implications for advanced nursing practice. Master's prepared nurses are clearly in the best possible position to facilitate the movement of clients through the health care delivery system without compromising on quality because they are prepared to provide complex multifaceted care in a wide variety of settings ranging from a research-oriented comprehensive medical center to a single occupant dwelling in a tiny rural community.

Societal Influences

A societal development that has been a driving force for requiring more master's prepared nurses is the population's emerging orientation toward wellness and self-care. Another development is the increasing emphasis on the need for more home care nursing and health services. Society, the health care industry, and state and federal governments now recognize that it is master's prepared nurse practitioners who can provide health promotion, health assessment, and health education programs to individuals and groups in primary care settings. They can also provide these services, as well as health restoration and management services to clients in their homes or in extended-care facilities.

DEVELOPMENT OF THE MASTER'S PROGRAM

The Terminal Degree

Development in the nature of master's-level nursing programs paralleled societal, technological, economic, and demographic developments with two unique features. One was that most people in the 1950s and 1960s viewed the master's degree in nursing as a terminal degree. This was because graduate nursing was a new development in the academic community and because there were so few baccalaureate-prepared nurses from which to draw and virtually no doctoral nursing programs in the country. The perception of master's programs in nursing as the terminal degree led to the programs being lengthier and more demanding than most other master's programs.

Role Preparation and Advanced Clinical Preparation

The other unique feature was a constant state of flux and uncertainty about program focus. Specifically, a review of the historical development of master's programs in nursing shows that in the 1950s and 1960s most programs emphasized role preparation rather than advanced clinical preparation. Typical curricular options for students during that period were nursing administration or nursing education. The clinical nursing courses that were available were minimal and usually had a strong medical orientation. A few programs required a clinical minor but in many programs clinical courses were only available for elective credit. This phenomenon is not surprising since the development of nursing theory and of advanced nursing practice models were in their embryonic states. What was encouraging, however, was the fact that hospitals were beginning to see the need for nursing administrators who possessed knowledge about management theory and who could apply this theory to nursing practice. Those associated with nursing education were also becoming convinced that nursing students needed to be educated by nurses who possessed expertise in higher education principles. As more and more nurses pursued master's degrees in fields related to nursing a shift from role preparation to clinical preparation began to occur.

During the late 1960s and early 1970s the number of master's programs in nursing increased significantly, the role of the clinical specialist and the nurse practitioner emerged, and clinical preparation literally replaced role preparation in master's programs in nursing. The four most common specialties in the early history of clinical specialization were medical/surgical nursing, psychiatric nursing, maternal/child health nursing, and community health nursing. The development of nursing theory, an increase in the number of nurse researchers, and a continuing shift in the health care delivery system created the need for other specialties and subspecialties; the demand for qualified associate and baccalaureate degree program faculty who had an advanced clinical knowledge base and finely honed clinical practice skills accelerated markedly as the number of associate degree programs skyrocketed and the number of baccalaureate degrees increased significantly. During that period of associate degree and baccalaureate program proliferation, however, the shift from role preparation to advanced clinical preparation was so complete that nurse educators had little or no teaching expertise and clinical nurse specialists had little or no leadership/management expertise.

By the late 1970s the pendulum took another turn. Role preparation reappeared. But because the workplace demands placed upon master's prepared nurses in both education and practice settings were so great and because, at least in some quarters, the master's degree was still viewed as the terminal degree for nurses, program content remained extremely heavy and program length tended to be significantly longer than other master's programs offered at the same institution. Then another phenomenon began to occur that brought a new perspective to master's level programming. That phenomenon was the burgeoning development of doctoral programs in nursing.

CONCLUSION

In 1965 there were four doctoral nursing programs in the United States. By 1975 there were 12, by 1985 there were 36 and in 1987 the number is nearing 50. Clearly the master's degree is no longer viewed as the terminal degree for nurses. Concurrent with programmatic development at the doctoral level has been the reexamination of program requirements and expectations at the master's level. It is now a widely accepted fact that master's level preparation of independent nurse researchers, nurse educators for senior colleges and universities, or nurse administrators for complex health care organizations or for educational nursing programs is unrealistic and inappropriate. What is realistic and also highly responsive to societal needs is to prepare at the master's level nurses who possess advanced nursing knowledge and clinical practice skills in a specialized area of practice and who also possess the educational, managerial, and research skills inherent in the role of the clinical specialist and/or practitioner. As Ginzberg and others point out, master's prepared nurses must possess advanced nursing knowledge and clinical expertise; however, that preparation alone is inadequate to function effectively in the modern health care system (Ginzberg, 1987; Sullivan, 1986; Cleland, 1984).

What appears to be emerging now are master's programs that are more reasonable in length. Appropriately, their primary focus is clinical, with support courses and learning activities designed to facilitate the development of appropriate research, management, and teaching competencies. These curricular trends and the shift in content inherent in them are very clearly reflected in NLN's latest (1987) edition of *Characteristics of Master's Education in Nursing*. Approved by the membership of the National League for Nursing's Council of Baccalaureate and Higher Degree Programs at NLN's 1987 biennial convention, these characteristics are presented here in their entirety because they are a compelling and encouraging statement about the current quality and relevance of master's program in nursing.

> Master's education in nursing prepares graduates for advanced nursing practice who function in roles such as clinical specialists, nurse practitioners, administrators, and educators. The graduates practice in a variety of settings, provide leadership in specialty areas and initiate collaborative and consultative relationships with others for the purpose of improving nursing and health care

and influencing health policy....Graduate preparation for advanced practice in nursing encompasses both generalized and specialized areas of study. Preparation for advanced practice in nursing should address societal needs for nursing services and should be broad enough in scope to enable persons so prepared to serve in a variety of settings and locations...Master's education in nursing includes advanced role preparation as well as advanced clinical preparation. The relationship between clinical and role preparation varies, depending on the primary focus of the program. When advanced clinical preparation is the focus, theory for advanced roles in nursing is essential. When advanced role preparation is the focus, clinical theory appropriate to the advance role is essential. Regardless of the primary focus, opportunity for advanced practice will incorporate a synthesis of both the advanced clinical and advanced role components. (NLN Council of Baccalaureate and Higher Degree Programs, *Characteristics of Master's Education in Nursing,* 1987).

These characteristics reflect both the current status of and the future directions for nursing education programs at the master's level. They reflect the profession's responsiveness to societal needs for practicing nurses with an advanced specialized knowledge base and related practice skills. They also reflect nursing's continuing emergence as an academic discipline in its own right, with its own theoretical foundations, and with its own intelligent system for educating nurses at the graduate level. It appears that a proper balance has finally been struck within the context of master's programs in nursing—a balance between what is master's-level content and what is doctoral-level content, a balance between master's programs in nursing and master's programs in other fields, a balance between nursing content and support or cognate content within the programs themselves, and, most importantly, a balance between what can and should be achievable at the master's level and our performance expectations from graduates of these programs.

As a dynamic profession at the heart of the health care delivery system, nursing has been and must continue to be responsive to societal, governmental, technological, economic, educational, professional, and demographic shifts and developments as these occur, bearing in mind as we do so that neither society, nor our students are well served when we expect our master's prepared nurses "to be all things to all people." Rather we must bring a proper perspective to bear on the relationship between societal needs and educational realities. When that perspective is operationalized all concerned parties will be well served, the system for the education of nurses at all levels will be clarified, and the continued advancement of our profession will be assured. It is encouraging and accurate to conclude from this historical review that the clear and compelling trend in master's level nursing programs is a proper blend between relevance and realism. It is incumbent upon all those associated with graduate nursing education to see that this blend is further fostered and facilitated so that bright and energetic persons are attracted to these programs in sufficient numbers to meet the health and nursing needs of the society we are committed to serve.

REFERENCES

Cleland, V. (1984). An articulated model for preparing nursing administrators. *The Journal of Nursing Administration,* October, 23–31.

Ginzberg, E. (1987). New economic climate breeds new market. *Nursing & Health Care, 8* (3), 139.

Institute of Medicine. (1983). *Nursing and nursing education: Public policies and private actions.* Washington, DC: National Academy Press.

National League for Nursing. (1987). *Characteristics of master's education in nursing* (3rd ed.). Council of Baccalaureate and Higher Degree Programs. New York: Author.

Spitzer, R. B., & Davivier, M. (1987). Nursing in the 1990s: Expanding opportunities. *Nursing Administration Quarterly, 11* (2), 55–61.

Sullivan, T. (1986). Promoting partnership: Education, service and specialization. In *Patterns in specialization: Challenge to the curriculum* (pp. 7–13). New York: National League for Nursing.

United States Public Health Service. (1963). *Toward quality in nursing: Needs and goals.* Report of the Surgeon General's Consultant Group on Nursing. Washington, DC: U.S. Government Printing Office.

4 THE RESEARCH COMPONENT OF GRADUATE NURSING PROGRAMS: THE ACQUISITION OF COMPETENCE

Theresa Sharp, EdD, RN
Sylvia E. Hart, PhD, RN

Among the salient issues in graduate nursing education today is that of research competence—at what level should it be acquired, how much competence is needed at the various levels, and what is the relationship of the research component to the overall curriculum. In recent years nursing research has become highly visible. There are now many high quality nursing research textbooks available that are authored by nurses. Several highly regarded professional journals publish only nursing research. There is a widespread consensus reflected in the nursing literature that the quantity and quality of nursing research has increased significantly since 1950. Tangible proof that nursing research is recognized and respected occured recently with the passage of Public Law 99-158, which provided for the establishment of a National Center for Nursing Research.

However, as prolific as nursing research activity has become, the precise nursing research competencies needed by nurses with graduate degrees have not been precisely defined or described. Therefore, the focus of this chapter is nursing research competence and its acquisition within the context of graduate education. Four questions are discussed: What is nursing research? Why is it important? What kinds of competencies are needed by the professional nurse to conduct or participate in nursing research? Where and how are these competencies acquired? The chapter is concluded with a statement concerning differences in competencies achieved at two levels of graduate education in nursing (i.e., master's level and doctor of philosophy level) and how graduate nurse educators can facilitate the development of research competencies in their students.

WHAT IS NURSING RESEARCH?

Research is the use of scientific inquiry or empirical study to discover or generate new knowledge. "Research usually is associated with university education, and interest and commitment to research are inextricably related to a learning climate in which scholarly inquiry is valued" (Polit & Hungler, 1983, p. 4). The common theme among the discussions of nursing research in the nursing literature over the last four decades is that research is a systematic process by which we gain new knowledge. Nursing research is a process of scientific inquiry that generates scientific knowledge and the incorporation of that knowledge into practice. "Nursing research includes studies relevant to the diagnosis and treatment of human responses to actual or potential health problems. As such, nursing research covers scientific inquiry into fundamental biomedical and behavioral processes relevant to nursing and investigations relating to nursing interventions in patient care" (Merritt, 1986, p. 84).

In a presentation at the International Nursing Research Conference in Edmonton, Alberta, Canada in 1986, Hockey defined nursing research as "an attempt to extend the scientific knowledge base in any area of work for which nurses are predominantly and appropriately responsible" (p. 20). Sound nursing judgment and ethical consideration of clients are necessary ingredients of all nursing research. Nurses have a responsibility to be knowledgeable about the research process so that they can intelligently participate, or decline to participate, in research being conducted by others (Bush, 1985).

Research encompasses generation of knowledge, dissemination of knowledge, and utilization of knowledge. "Empirical, or scientific, knowledge encompasses descriptions, explanations, and predictions about observable phenomena that can be extrapolated beyond the samples used to develop the knowledge." In nursing this kind of knowledge is tested by basic, applied, and clinical research. Dissemination of knowledge obviously presupposes generation of knowledge and involves the presentation of research findings at conferences, publication of research reports in books, journals, monographs, and incorporation of research findings in textbooks, lectures, seminar discussions, and various media forms. Utilization of knowledge includes using the knowledge in clinical practice and use of research findings by researchers (Fawcett, 1985).

Traditionally, three types of nursing research have been identified as basic, applied, and clinical research. Basic research, also called theoretical or pure research, provides a general understanding of phenomena (Fawcett, 1984). Basic research generates and tests scientific theories about phenomena, whereas applied research tests the practical limits of scientific knowledge developed by basic research, and applied research typically employs the empirical methods of correlational and experimental designs. Clinical research studies the effects of applying scientific knowledge in the practice setting and may include use of empirical methods of clinical experiments or clinical trials (Fawcett, 1985).

The Cabinet on Nursing Research of the American Nurses' Association has published a document entitled *Directions for Nursing Research: Toward the Twenty-first Century*. In this publication the Cabinet identifies the focus of nursing research. "Nursing research generates knowledge about health and health promotion in individuals and families and knowledge about the influence of social and physical environments on health. Nursing research also addresses the care of persons who are acutely or chronically ill, disabled, or dying, as well as the care of their families. In addition, nursing research studies therapeutic actions that minimize the negative effects of illness by enhancing the abilities of individuals and families to respond to actual or potential health problems. Nursing research also emphasizes the generation of knowledge about (1) systems that effectively and efficiently deliver health care, (2) the profession and its historical development, (3) ethical guidelines for the delivery of nursing services, and (4) systems that effectively and efficiently prepare nurses to fulfill the profession's current and future social mandate (*Directions for Nursing Research: Toward the Twenty-first Century*, 1987). This focus statement spans the depth and scope of professional nursing as it exists in current times, and mandates acquisition of research competence by graduates of baccalaureate, master's, and doctoral degree programs.

WHY IS NURSING RESEARCH IMPORTANT?

Nursing research is important because it yields the knowledge that legitimizes the science of nursing. Nursing research is important because application of the knowledge derived from research contributes to the improvement of nursing practice, health care, and health promotion. Nursing research is important because it can add a continuous new vitality to the discipline from within the discipline and from outside the discipline through multidisciplinary research collaboration. Nursing research is important because it can provide the nursing profession with new methods, alternatives, or systems for achieving stronger professional autonomy, for more cost-effective nursing and health care delivery and for scientifically supported professional accountability. Finally, nursing research is important because, as stated by the ANA Cabinet on Research, "The future of nursing practice and, ultimately, the future of health care in this country depend on nursing research designed to constantly generate an up-to-date, organized body of knowledge" (*Directions for Nursing Research: Toward the Twenty-first Century*, 1987).

Stevenson has written that "research flourishes best in environments that nourish, encourage, and support it. . . Considerable progress has been made in the development of nursing research in the United States since 1950" (1987, pp. 60, 63). Larson wrote in 1984 that "interest in nursing research has, probably for the first time, been expressed by the entire scientific community as a result of approval in 1983 of a House of Representatives' bill proposing an Institute of Nursing within the National Institutes of Health (NIH)" (p. 131). This tangible monument to the importance of nursing research was realized when a $16 million budget for The National Center for Nursing Research (NCNR) was authorized under the Health Research Extension Act of 1985, P.L. 99–158 (Merritt, 1986, pp. 84, 85; Stevenson, 1987, p. 60).

RESEARCH COMPETENCE

What kind of research competence do graduate-prepared nurses need? Hockey stated that "one has to establish one's competence by means of credentials" and "proven competence can do a great deal to negotiate frontiers between professional as well as academic disciplines" (1986, pp. 22, 23). Cronewett (1986) addressed the expectations for the competence of those who do research: "No other profession has the same expectations for the conduct of research that nursing has placed on nondoctorally prepared people. Just as becoming an expert clinician requires knowledge, practice, and experience, so, too, are those elements required to become a competent researcher. Although the profession has been concerned with identifying minimum competency levels for clinical practice, we have yet to devote the same energy to identifying what knowledge, skills, and experience are necessary to be considered competent to conduct research" (p. 11). Stevenson discussed the increased interest in nursing research and alluded to competence of nursing researchers in a 1987 article. She discussed the historical perspective of nursing research spanning the decades from the 1950s into the 1980s and made this erudite observation: "The challenges before us are not less than in 1950. Rather, they are greater than ever before...Now nursing is in the limelight. The science produced by nurses is being critiqued by members of other health disciplines...The past is prologue; the challenge for scientific excellence now sits squarely on nursing's shoulders" (p. 63).

What is it about research and the nature of nursing research that warrants a focus on competence and a challenge for excellence from nursing's scientists? Research in general is a complex process. Nursing research is uniquely complex because of the unique nature of nursing. Hockey alluded to that uniqueness in 1986 with this opinion: "Nurse researchers must gain sufficient self-confidence to develop new and creative relationships with other disciplines, if only to explore the utility of their approaches to the study of nursing and to attempt an appropriate unique mix of research approaches to match that of nursing itself" (p. 23).

At a time when the focus on professional accountability is at an all-time high and increasing, and at a time when there is increased national focus on nursing research, the nursing profession is both challenged and pressed to ensure that its researchers and its consumers of nursing research are competent.

Webster's Third New International Dictionary of the English Language, Unabridged defines competent as "possessed of or characterized by marked or sufficient aptitude, skill, strength or knowledge...possessed of knowledge, judgment, strength, or skill needed to perform an indicated action" (p. 463). *Black's Law Dictionary* provides a legal viewpoint when it defines competent as "duly qualified; answering all requirements; having sufficient ability or authority; possessing the requisite natural or legal qualifications" (1979, p. 257). The same law dictionary defined "skill" as "practical and familiar knowledge of the principles and processes of an art, science, or trade, combined with the ability to apply them in practice in a proper and approved manner and with readiness and dexterity" (p. 1244).

Six important research competencies are presented here beginning with the simplest and concluding with the most complex. First, the nurse must be a competent and intelligent consumer and utilizer of research findings. Skills associated with this competence include critical analysis and appropriate utilization of tested research findings in clinical practice. A second level of competence is the ability to identify researchable clinical problems. These problems can be referred to qualified nurse researchers for comprehensive investigation. A slightly higher level of competence is the ability to function as an authentic interdisciplinary and intradisciplinary collaborator in data collection and analysis.

A fourth nursing research competence is dissemination of research findings through through publications, presentations, or other forms of professional dialogue. A fifth research competence is the ability to test new applications of existing research findings to nursing practice. The ability to develop and test nursing theory is the sixth research competency that some nurses must possess if nursing is to be unarguably recognized and acknowledged as an authentic scientific discipline.

Baccalaureate Degree Programs

The competencies that are described in the preceding paragraph are progressively developed in baccalaureate, master's and doctor of philosophy nursing programs. The baccalaureate-prepared nurse should know and understand research language and the research process. He or she should be able to critique research studies, and to function as an intelligent consumer and utilizer of research findings in his or her practice. These competencies are reflected in the NLN accreditation criteria and guidelines for baccalaureate nursing programs.

Criterion 26 states that "The research process and its contribution to nursing are included in the curriculum." The guidelines for interpretation of this criterion are: (1) Content and instructional activities are designed to assist the student in attaining the ability to evaluate research for the applicability of its findings to nursing action; and (2) Content and instructional activities are designed to assist the student in attaining the ability to identify research problems in nursing practice. (*Self-Study Manual: Guidelines for Preparation of the Self-Study Report,* 1984, p. 44).

The 1980 ANA Commission on Nursing Education's report to the ANA House of Delegates contained the following language concerning the investigative guidelines for the baccalaureate level. These guidelines are highly compatible with the NLN research criterion and guidelines.

The baccalaureate prepared nurse

1. Reads, interprets, and evaluates research for applicability to nursing practice.

2. Identifies nursing problems that need to be investigated and participates in the implementation of scientific studies.

3. Uses nursing practice as a means of gathering data for refining and extending practice.

4. Applies established findings of nursing and other health-related research to nursing practice.

5. Shares research findings with colleagues. (*Guidelines for the Investigative Function of Nurses,* 1981).

Baccalaureate programs vary widely in their methodology for incorporating this content into the curriculum. Some programs have separate courses in research, statistics, and computer applications. Others integrate all of the content into several or all of their nursing courses.

Master's Degree Programs

The research content at the baccalaureate level is discussed here because it serves as the foundation upon which master's level research competence is built. There is general agreement that master's prepared nurses should be able to assume an active collaborative role in such research activities as data collection and analysis. The master's prepared nurse's ability to critique research studies and to apply research findings to clinical practice problems needs to be finely honed.

The National League for Nursing's criterion relative to research competence at the master's level is criterion 32 which reads: "The curriculum provides for the acquisition of knowledge and skills in scientific inquiry, the ability to validate and extend research findings in practice; and the ability to evaluate nursing theory appropriate for advanced professional practice."

The guidelines for interpretation of this criterion are:

Through course work and clinical practice, students are provided the opportunity to:
- Derive from nursing theory and other theory, propositions which can be tested in practice.
- Analyze research findings and test their application in practice.
- Derive from their practice generalizations/propositions which can be tested systematically.

(*Self-Study Manual: Guidelines for Preparation of the Self-Study Report*, 1984, p. 50)

Mastery of the research principles reflected in these guidelines can be achieved in a variety of ways. Methods used include, but are not limited to, such learning activities as the generation of research papers, literature reviews, oral and written presentations or research reports, case studies, research-oriented clinical assignments, or a thesis or project.

The ANA Commission on Nursing Education has identified guidelines for the investigative function at the master's degree level. These guidelines are highly compatible with NLN accreditation criteria and guidelines and are stated as follows:

1. Analyzes and reformulates nursing practice problems so that scientific knowledge and scientific methods can be used to find solutions.

2. Enhances the quality and clinical relevance of nursing research by providing expertise in clinical problems and by providing knowledge about the way in which these clinical services are delivered.

3. Facilitates investigations of problems in clinical settings through such activities as contributing to a climate supportive of investigative activities, collaborating with others in investigations and enhancing nursing's access to clients and data.

4. Conducts investigations for the purpose of monitoring the quality of the practice of nursing in a clinical setting.

5. Assists others to apply scientific knowlege in nursing practice.

A typical master's program in nursing includes a separate research course, statistics content, computer science content, and a formalized research "exercise" that is called either a thesis or a project. Upon completion of a master's program graduates must possess a repetoire of research competencies that become integrated into their advanced clinical practice as well as into their teaching or management roles.

Doctoral Degree Programs

Prior to the mid-1970s four programs in the United States offered doctoral preparation with a nursing major. Although the number of doctoral programs has increased markedly since the early 1970s, the need for doctorally prepared nurses remains "staggering" and "the pressure to fill the need for increased numbers of doctorally prepared nurses threatens the quality of nursing science, its researach programs, and the viability of doctoral education in nursing" (Holzemer, 1987, p. 111). In June 1987 there were 44 doctoral programs in nursing in the United States. The major focus of the discussion about research competence at the doctoral level will be confined to the doctor of philosophy programs since the doctorate of philosophy is the nationally recognized research degree. However, a brief review of the various doctoral degrees in nursing currently being conferred is also presented since all of these programs do include a research component.

In 1986 Snyder-Halpern reported that research comparing different types of doctoral programs in nursing has not been done (p. 360). The degrees awarded at the doctoral level in nursing include: The Doctor of Philosophy (PhD), The Doctor of Nursing Science (DNS, DSN, DNSc), and The Doctor of Education (EdD). In 1978, Downs described the three types of programs that currently comprise the doctoral degree structure in nursing. "The PhD degree is described as a research degree which implies an ability to carry out meaningful research, discover new knowledge, and usually indicates appropriate preparation for university teaching. The DNS, DSN, DNSc degrees constitute a professional degree which is described as the 'highest university award given in a particular field in recognition of completion of academic preparation for professional practice.' The EdD degree is described as a generic degree that emphasizes scholarship and research primarily in education at the doctoral level in a manner that is more applied than that found in PhD degree programs" (Snyder-Halpern, 1986, p. 358). A slightly different categorization has been presented by Holzemer in his discussion of the assessment of quality of doctoral education in nursing spanning the years 1979–1984. According to Holzemer, doctoral education in nursing has focused on two primary degree routes, namely "the professional doctorate" and the doctor of philosophy in nursing. Holzemer states that "professional doctoral programs emphasize the application of research findings to clinical nursing. The programs that emphasize more basic research award the Doctor of Philosophy in nursing" (1987, p. 111). The ANA has developed two sets of guidelines for the research competencies expected from "practice-oriented" and "research-oriented" doctoral programs. Developed by the ANA Commission on Nursing Education in 1980, the guidelines are:

The graduate of a practice-oriented doctoral program

1. Provides leadership for the integration of scientific knowledge with other sources of knowledge for the advancement of practice.

2. Conducts investigations to evaluate the contribution of nursing activities to the well-being of clients.

3. Develops methods to monitor the quality of the practice of nurs-

ing in a clinical setting and to evaluate contributions of nursing activities to the well-being of clients.

The graduate of a research-oriented doctoral program

1. Develops theoretical explanations of phenomena relevant to nursing by empirical research and analytical processes.

2. Uses analytical and empirical methods to discover ways to modify or extend existing scientific knowledge so that it is relevant to nursing.

3. Develops methods for scientific inquiry of phenomena relevant to nursing (*Guidelines for the Investigative Function of Nurses,* 1981).

Research Activities of Master's Degree and Doctoral Degree Nurses

In 1985 Fawcett presented a typology of nursing research activities according to educational preparation. In that article, Fawcett discusses the ANA guidelines. Her interpretation is that the ANA guidelines indicate that doctorally prepared nurses and, to a lesser extent, master's prepared nurses are responsible for the generation of nursing research. "Graduates of research-oriented doctoral programs are prepared to conduct basic, applied, and clinical research. Graduates of practice-oriented doctoral programs are prepared to conduct applied and clinical research. Graduates of Master's degree programs are prepared to conduct clinical research, especially the clinical trials needed to determine the quality and efficacy of nursing practice" (p. 76). While Fawcett's distinctions between master's and doctoral degree programs is currently operational, the research competency distinctions among the various kinds of doctoral programs is less clear in actual practice.

In any event the research-oriented doctorally prepared nurse scientist is prepared to discover and extend knowledge relevant to nursing. "Generally, a nursing program is based on a philosophy which serves as a foundation for the curriculum" (Arnold & Sherwen, 1986, p. 327). The research-oriented doctoral degree curriculum, therefore, should reflect a belief system that emphasizes a comprehensive knowledge of the research process and the active participation in a variety of research activities, investigations, and scientific inquiries related to nursing. This kind of doctoral degree program typically includes advanced content in research design and methodology, advanced statistics, computer science, theoretical foundations and theory development including content specific to development of nursing science and opportunity for independent scientific investigations. Central to a legitimate doctorate of philosophy degree program is the development, completion, and defense of a dissertation. The doctorate of philosophy prepared nurse, in other words, must possess the same repetoire of research competencies that are evidenced by his or her colleagues in other academic disciplines with the ability to discover, advance and disseminate new knowledge as the critical and central behavior that must be acquired.

Clearly scientific inquiry is and must be an integral part of graduate study in nursing. At the master's level, programs must be designed to ensure that the graduate will be able to analyze theoretical and empirical knowledge from the sciences, humanities, and nursing for its applicability to provision of nursing care for defined populations. Students need the opportunity to develop and demonstrate knowledge of the research process through course work that includes advanced nursing content, research methodology, advanced statistics, with opportunities to do research critiques, conduct investigations, participate in research projects, write research papers and present research findings.

Research-oriented doctoral programs should ensure that graduates have advanced knowledge in the research process and can demonstrate the ability to independently conduct scientific investigations. In fact, the primary purpose of the research-oriented doctoral program in nursing is to prepare nurse scientists who have the advanced knowledge and research competence to discover and extend knowledge relevant to nursing. Terminal research competencies for graduates of these programs include the ability to test and/or generate knowledge from the biological and behavioral sciences for application to advanced clinical nursing practice; test and/or generate nursing theory to advance clinical nursing practice; design, conduct or direct clinically oriented research designed to improve nursing and health care; and analyze and judge research for its incorporation in nursing.

The continued development of nursing as a scientific academic discipline is heavily dependent upon the collective research competence of the members of the profession. It is therefore incumbent upon all who are associated with graduate nursing education to continue to develop these competencies in themselves and in their students. The profession's demonstrated commitment to meeting the health and nursing needs of society is made visible each time new knowledge is discovered.

REFERENCES

Arnold, J. M., & Sherwen, L. N. (1986). Belief systems which influence research in nursing: Implications for preparing future investigators. *Journal of Nursing Education, 25,* 325–327.

Black's law dictionary (5th ed.). (1979). St. Paul, Minnesota: West Publishing.

Bush, C. T. (1985). *Nursing research.* Reston, Virginia: Reston Publishing Co., Inc.

Cronenwett, L. R. (1986). Research reflections: The research role of the clinical nurse specialist. *The Journal of Nursing Administration, 16,* 10–11.

Directions for nursing research: Toward the twenty-first century. (1985). Kansas City, Missouri: American Nurses' Association, Cabinet on Nursing Research.

Fawcett, J. (1985). A typology of nursing research activities according to education preparation. *Journal of Professional Nursing, 1,* 75–78.

Fawcett, J. (1984). Another look at utilization of nursing research. *Image: The Journal of Nursing Scholarship, XVI,* 59–62.

Gove, P. B. (Ed.). (1971). *Webster's third new international dictionary of the English language, Unabridged.* Springfield, Massachusetts: G. & C. Merriam.

Guidelines for the investigative function of nurses. (1981). Kansas City, Missouri: American Nurses' Association, Commission on Nursing Research.

Hockey, L. (1986, May). Frontiers of nursing research–Real or imagined? In S. M. Stinson, J. C. Kerr, P. Giovannetti, P. A. Field, & J. MacPhail (Eds.). *New frontiers in nursing research.* Proceedings of the International Nursing Research Conference, University of Alberta, Edmonton.

Holzemer, W. L. (1987). Doctoral education in nursing: An assessment of quality, 1979–1984. *Nursing Research, 36,* 111–116.

Larson, E. (1984). The current status of nursing research. *Nursing Forum, XXI,* 131–134.

Merritt, D. M. (1986). The national center for nursing research. *Image: Journal of Nursing Scholarship, 18,* 84–85.

Polit, D. F., & Hungler, B. P. (1983). *Nursing research: Principles and methods* (2nd ed.). Philadelphia: J. B. Lippincott.

Self-study manual: Guidelines for preparation of the self-study report. (1984). New York: National League for Nursing, Council of Baccalaureate and Higher Degree Programs.

Snyder-Halpern, R. (1986). Doctoral programs in nursing: An examination of curriculum similarities and differences. *Journal of Nursing Education, 25,* 358–365.

Stevenson, J. S. (1987). Forging a research discipline. *Nursing Research, 36,* 60–64.

5 MODELS FOR DOCTORAL PROGRAMS: FIRST PROFESSIONAL DEGREE OR TERMINAL DEGREE?

Patricia R. Forni, PhD, RN, FAAN

Nursing's quest for professional stature and disciplinary status, with roots in the training schools of nineteenth-century England and America, is closely tied to the struggle of women for achievement of equality and worth. The very name of the profession, nursing, connotes assistance, succor, nurturance—all feminine traits. The term nurse is derived from these traits and is a title that has come to be associated with a primarily female group. It is interesting to note that until the turn of the century that titles of bachelor's and master's degrees for women graduates were regarded as lacking in propriety, and alternative titles of mistress, maid, or sister were used.

Many of nursing's problems continue to emanate from its feminine orientation. It has been said that we suffer from a lack of self-esteem and that we have an over romanticized view of science (Matarazzo, 1971). In more recent times as nursing education has become a part of higher education, the acquisition of degrees has enhanced society's regard for, and image of, nursing. However, nursing's ascendence of the educational ladder has also been accompanied by society's and the profession's confusion regarding educational models, role delineation, practice parameters, and titling issues.

In this chapter, contemporary models of doctoral education in nursing will be examined to assess where they may be leading as we approach the twenty-first century and continue to pursue our dual quests for professional equality and achievement.

HISTORY OF DOCTORAL EDUCATION AND THE ORGIN OF DEGREES IN THE UNITED STATES

The history of doctoral education in the United States has been well-documented by Spurr (1970), Berelson (1960), Rashdall (1936), and others.

45

Doctoral education in the United States originated in the second half of the nineteenth century and was patterned after the German system. A large number of Americans educated in German research-oriented universities influenced the development of a similar model in the United States. The first Doctor of Philosophy (Ph.D.) as an earned degree was awarded by Yale University in 1861. One of the first three scholars to receive the degree in that year, James Morris Whiton, studied without a professor for two years but passed exams and produced a six-page thesis. The degree requirements at that time were three-fold: two years of post-baccalaureate study, a thesis, and a final examination.

The founding of Johns Hopkins University as a graduate school in 1876 marked the beginning of the American university. Hopkins has played a major role in the development of graduate education and the PhD. Hopkins, known for high standards, adopted policies and practices which were emulated by other universities. In 1881, the length of time between the bachelor's degree and the doctorate was increased from two to three years. A graduate academic council was formed in 1883 to monitor quality; in the next year subordinate studies were increased to two years from one. In 1885 an outline was adopted for the thesis with the recommendation that it be typewritten; one copy was required for the library. Two years later, reading examinations in French and German were added, along with the requirements of an official adviser and two external examiners for reading the thesis.

By 1896 students had come to play a strong role in influencing the quality of programs. At the 1896 convention of the Federation of Graduate Clubs, students made four sweeping recommendations which essentially remain with us today: (1) the reqirement of a bachelor's degree or its equivalent; (2) a residency requirement of two years at least, one of which should be on campus; (3) an examination; and (4) a thesis, based upon original research, acceptable to the department or major professor.

Following this, two organizations, the Association of American Universities and the National Association of State Universities, futher strengthened the requirements of the PhD. Prior to World War I they had established that the period of study be three years, at least one of which should be spent in residence at the university. Subsequently other changes took place to strengthen the PhD. These changes included eliminating the practice of awarding the PhD as an honorary degree, extending the degree to applied fields, and lengthening the period of enrollment to four to five years.

More recent changes have included reductions in the foreign language requirement, additional graduate level coursework, emphasis on early qualifying exams, and in some cases microfilming, rather than printing of the dissertation (Spurr, 1970).

Origin of Degrees

The terms doctor and master originated in the early Middle Ages at Bologna and Paris, sites of the two original universities. These titles were conferred on students who had successfully completed their course of studies and had been admitted to the teaching faculty (guilds). While Bologna was the center of learning in civil and canon law, Paris was the center of study for the arts. The English system that developed at Oxford and Cambridge adopted the French use of master. The German use of doctor was adopted from Bologna. The title of professor was used interchangeably with the other two at the time. Eventually the titles of master and doctor came to represent a degree rather than an office, whereas the title of professor came to represent senior rank as a teacher.

Because the system of undergraduate education in the United States was based upon the English college model, the Bachelor of Arts degree was the only earned degree awarded for over two hundred years following the founding of Harvard College in 1636. The Bachelor of Science degree was introduced in 1851, also by Harvard. From the founding of Harvard to around the Civil War, a pro forma Master of Arts (MA) degree was awarded to those who paid their fees for three or so years and remained in good standing. The *in cursu* ("as a matter of course") degree was later replaced by the earned *pro meritis* MA first awarded in 1859 at the University of Michigan (Spurr, 1970).

Berelson (1960, p. 10) summarizes the evolution of higher education by saying, "A graduate school based on the German model was placed on top of an undergraduate college based on the English model, and several people believe that this arrangement has plagued the system ever since."

Professional Degrees

The doctorate as a professional degree originated in the Middle Ages in the original learned professions of medicine, law, and theology. Since then professional degrees have been established in many fields. The EdD (doctorate in education) as a professional degree was established in 1920 at Harvard University and was awarded by the School of Education rather than the graduate school. Several reasons are offered as to why the EdD was initiated: (1) the admission requirements of the school of education can be less stringent than those of the graduate school, (2) the foreign language requirements can be avoided, (3) a range of projects can be substituted for the dissertation, (4) an expository work rather than one based upon original research can be done, and (5) a reduction in time to earn the degree can be achieved (Spurr, 1970).

The Doctor of Arts degree (DA) as a teaching degree was revived in the early 1960s. The Council of Graduate Schools in the United States issued a statement on "The Doctor of Arts Degree" in 1970. The program characteristics were delineated then as: (1) formal course work primarily in the subject matter to be taught; (2) specified coursework dealing with learning, higher education, and faculty roles; (3) a teaching internship; (4) familiarity with current pedagogical developments; (5) ability to apply the latest techniques to teaching; and (6) a "suitable written thesis" on an area in the subject field.

Degrees for Women

Until the latter half of the nineteenth century it was considered improper to award academic degrees to women. Hence, institutions in the United States went to great lengths not to award a bachelor's degree to young women graduates. Catherine Beecher, a pioneer in higher education for women, wrote in 1835 that, "it certainly is in very bad taste, and would provoke needless ridicule and painful notoriety" (Eells & Haswell, 1960, p. 37). As this was apparently a widely held view, many institutions adopted as the appropriate title for female graduates, Mistress, Maid, or Sister although the latter title did not gain wide acceptance. In 1856 Beaver College, Pennsylvania conferred two degrees, the Mistress of Liberal Arts and the Mistress of English Literature. Two other practices adopted at the time were the use of Graduate and Laureate as titles for female graduates. It appears that the designation of a different degree for women virtually disappeared in the last decade of the nineteenth century, but Burnett College, Tennessee awarded the Mistress degree as late as 1924.

In contrast, by 1958–59, of all degrees conferred in the United States, 11 percent of the doctoral degrees, 32 percent of the master's degrees, and 34 percent of the bachelor's degrees were earned by women (Eells and Haswell, 1960). By 1974, 20.5 percent of the doctoral degrees awarded in the United States were earned by women (National Research Council, 1978).

THE NATURE OF PROFESSIONAL EDUCATION

Brubacher (1962) traces the early origins of professional education to Roman times. Quintilian in his *Institues of Oratory* identified three components of professional education as we know it today. These were: (1) a knowledge base in one's subject matter, (2) a liberal education including knowledge of the society and culture in which one works, and (3) opportunity to practice in order to perfect one's skills.

The importance of a liberal education was further emphasized in the medieval university, where a "bachelor's degree was a prerequisite to professional training" (Brubacher, 1962, p. 52). The degree, however, was awarded at the beginning of the course of study rather than at the end as is now the case. The culmination of study was the awarding of the master's degree, which carried with it the license to teach. In other words, the student had become master.

The apprenticeship was an important part of professional training dating back to Greco-Roman times, but it was not until the Middle Ages that the relationship became one of student to professor rather than apprentice to master. Learning by apprenticeship was carried over into the nineteenth century, and professional education was characterized by learning by doing. Over time a change occured, whereby professors began handing down information through lectures and learning took place by listening to lectures rather than by doing. Eventually lectures were written and textbooks emerged. Thus, didactic learning became formalized.

The apprenticeship approach to education was dramatically changed when, at Johns Hopkins University, the medical internship was formalized as part of the medical training period. Several other measures were employed to elevate the medical profession to university rank. The teaching and practice of medicine began to draw on the basic sciences and the medical knowledge base was enlarged. Harvard made the bachelor's degree a requirement for entrance into medical school and raised tuition. This was considered a bold move at the time and it was predicted that enrollments would drop, a temporary prediction which held for a short time (Brubacher, 1962).

The defining of a field of education as a profession has been addressed by many. Flexner (1930), speaking on professions, wrote:

> How are we to distinguish professions that belong to universities from vocations that do not belong to them? The criteria are not difficult to discern. Professions are, as a matter of history and very rightly 'learned professions'; there are no unlearned professions. Unlearned professions—a contradiction in terms would be vocations, callings, or occupations. (p. 29)

HISTORICAL DEVELOPMENT OF THE DOCTORATE IN NURSING

The historical development of doctoral education for nurses has been chronicled by Grace (1978) and Murphy (1981), who traced the progress in periods of development. Grace (1978) considered the development in three steps; the first step was doctoral education *for* nurses in education and administration; the second was doctoral education *for* nurses in a second discipline in one of the basic or social sciences; and the third was doctoral education *in* nursing.

Murphy (1981) depicts phase one as that of preparation for functional specialists (1952–1959), phase two as that of nurse scientists (1960–1969), and phase three as that of doctorates in and of nursing (1970 to present). More recently Stevenson & Woods (1986) have described four generations of nurses with doctorates. From 1900 through 1940 the first generation was comprised of nurses with the EdD or other functional doctorates. The second (1940–1960) was the generation taking PhDs in the basic or social sciences with no nursing content. The third generation fell in the decade of the 1960s (1960–1970) and included the PhDs in basic sciences with a minor in nursing. The fourth and present generation (1970–present) is the one of the doctorate in nursing, PhD, or Doctor of Nursing Science (DNS). The next generation (2000 and beyond) is projected to be one of "greater specificity within nursing" and "formalized postdoctoral programs" (Stevenson & Woods, 1986, p. 8).

The number of doctoral programs in nursing has grown exponentially. In 1960 there were but four doctoral programs in nursing; in 1980 there were 21 (Grace, 1963); and in 1986 there were 45 (National League for Nursing, 1987). It is predicted that an additional 21 programs will be in operation by 1995 (Brodie, 1986).

The two earliest doctoral programs in nursing were initiated at Teachers College-Columbia University (TC) and New York University (NYU). Teachers College, which initiated the Doctor of Education (EdD) program in 1933, still offers it today. New York University initiated the EdD in 1934 and phased it out around 1960 at which time the PhD program was started (D. McGivern, personal communication, July 15, 1987). The next doctoral program to be initiated was the PhD at the University of Pittsburgh in 1954, followed by the DNS at Boston University in 1960, at the University of California-San Francisco in 1964, and at Catholic University in 1967 (Matarazzo & Abdellah, 1971).

The federal government played a significant role in the development of doctoral education in the United States. Starting in 1955 the United States Public Health Service awarded Special Predoctoral Research Fellowships directly to individual doctoral students. In the 1960s, the Nurse-Scientist Graduate Training Program was initiated. These awards were given to institutions with programs offering doctorates in a basic or social science with a minor in nursing (Matarazzo & Abdellah, 1971). In some cases the minor in nursing was not required.

In 1965 four nursing leaders discussed their views on approaches to doctoral preparation at a symposium held at Frances Payne Bolton School of Nursing, Case Western Reserve University. Their positions reflected the status of doctoral education of nurses at that time. They all concurred that the PhD was an appropriate degree for nurses, although they described different routes to attaining that end. Dr. Mary Tschudin spoke of the need for nursing to become a fully participating member of the university community. She said:

> For too long we have been remiss in not accepting our full responsibilities as members of the university family, we have been 'in' but not 'of' the university because we have not been prepared to participate in carrying out the full range of university functions. (1966, p. 50).

Dr. Tschudin described one route to the PhD for nurses—the nurse-scientist training program. In this approach nurses obtained a PhD in a science basic to nursing and a minor in nursing. At the University of Washington where she was then dean, the nurse-scientist program offered doctoral study in anthropology, microbiology, physiology, or sociology.

Dr. Hildegard Peplau (1966) recognized both the PhD and the professional doctorate as avenues for doctoral education in nursing. She advocated that a theoretical core of knowledge be developed for each clinical area and supported the idea of a PhD in clinical nursing.

Dr. Rozella Schlotfeldt (1966) took the position that nurses seeking doctoral education should do so in a field of fundamental knowledge such as biology, psychology, physiology, history, philosophy, and so forth. She likened this approach to that in medicine where physicians are at once doctors and scientists. She believed that nurses prepared in basic disciplines could apply their knowledge in nursing and contribute as scholars, researchers, educators, and administrators.

Dr. Martha Rogers (1966), as head of New York University's Department of Nurse Education, which offered a PhD in nursing at that time, spoke strongly in favor of this degree. In making a case for the PhD in nursing she used the analogy of the student who ultimately wished to be a clinical psychologist and asked whether such a student would take doctoral work in engineering or microbiology to achieve this end. Arguing against the position taken by Schlotfeldt, that nurses should attain PhDs in basic disciplines, she observed that nursing is not additive, but creative; therefore, "one simply does not take knowledges from a variety of different sources and say, "We'll add these together and somehow they will constitute nursing knowledge'" (1966, p. 78).

The common theme expressed by the four symposium speakers was that the PhD was the appropriate degree for nurses, but the speakers viewed the approaches for achieving it differently. One speaker also recognized the professional doctorate, the Doctor of Nursing Science (DNSc), as an appropriate degree. Matarazzo (1971, p. 81) in analyzing the symposium noted that, "The four symposium panelists met their charge well. They quickly dispensed with the EdD option by never mentioning it."

In 1971 the Division of Nursing, United States Public Health Service (USPHS), held an invitational conference on Future Directions of Doctoral Education for Nurses. Some noteworthy observations were made at the conference. Two principal reasons for nursing's reluctance to move ahead in the development of PhD programs in nursing were identified as nursing's self-concept and its romanticized view of science. Joseph Matarazzo, PhD, the conference chairperson and a non-nurse, chided the profession by saying:

> ...what the scientist does is the very antithesis of the nonsense... [nurses] write in their articles about the relationship between nursing and science. Nursing textbooks insist that science is orderly; that people are supposed to go through step one, step two, step three, step four. Science isn't like that. It doesn't follow well-established rules and principles. It is messy, unguided, untutored, personal, and biased. It is full of rage, anger, hostility and optimism. And it is fun. (1971, p. 11)

However, Matarozzo believed that nursing was ready to move ahead with development of the PhD in nursing far earlier than it did.

THE DOCTORATE AS THE FIRST PROFESSIONAL DEGREE

Models for doctoral programs: first professional degree or terminal degree? This provocative question has no clear-cut answer. The philosophy, goals, and mission of the nursing program should guide deliberations as to which doctoral model to follow. However, as we shall see the doctorate as the first professional degree was never conceived as a replacement for the terminal doctorate.

Newman (1975) advocated that the professional doctorate in nursing (the Doctor of Nursing degree) be offered as the first professional degree as a means of gaining recognition and authority for nursing.

The doctorate as the first professional degree, equivalent to the MD and offered as the ND, was first proposed by Scholtfeldt (1978). In the model she espoused, one fashioned after the medical model, nurses would be educated in a discipline outside of nursing at the baccalaureate level. This education would then form the basis for study in nursing at the postbaccalaureate level leading to the award of the doctor of nursing degree, the ND. Schlotfeldt (1978, p. 308) identified what she considered "two persisting flaws" in baccalaureate nursing programs at that time. One is the technical emphasis in the curriculum: students are required to learn to do prior to or concurrent with learning to know. The second deficiency derived from the faculty's not having responsibility for quality control of the clinical practicum setting. She saw the ND, offered in a health science center where nursing faculty would exercise control over the quality of care, as offering the means for eradicating the two flaws. Her position that nursing preparation should be at the postbaccalaureate level derived from her strong belief that this model, more than any other, would allow nursing to achieve full professional status.

The doctor of nursing model (the N. D.) was initiated in 1979 at Case Western Reserve University where it is flourishing today. However, the model has not caught on at other institutions, and the Frances Payne Bolton School of Nursing remains the only one in the country offering the degree in 1987. However, one other such program is in the planning stages.

In writing about "knowledge viewed in relation to professional skill" John Henry Newman in 1859 cited the scholar Dr. Edward Copleston:

> But the professional character is not the only one which a person engaged in a profession has to support. He is not always upon duty...As a friend, as a companion, as a citizen at large; in the connections of domestic life; in the improvement and embellishment of his leisure, he has a sphere of action, revolving if you please, within the sphere of his profession, but not clashing with it,

in which if he can show none of the advantages of an improved understanding, whatever may be his skill or proficiency in the other, he is no more than an ill-educated man. (p. 149)

More recent developments in higher education give strength to the position that the preparatory program in the profession should be at the postbaccalaureate level. I am referring to the renewed interest in and movement toward strengthening the undergraduate curriculum in four-year institutions of higher learning to include greater preparation for citizenship through a broadened liberal education.

The American Association of Colleges of Nursing received funding from the Pew Memorial Trust to carry out a project to define the components of education for professional nursing. A national panel directed the study, called *Essentials of College and University Education for Professional Nursing* (1986). The panel recommended education for professional nursing "so that the graduate will exhibit qualities of mind and character that are necessary to live a free and fulfilling life, act in the public interest locally and globally, and contribute to health care improvements and the nursing profession" (AACN, 1986, p. 4). To achieve this end the panel further recommended that the following seven values were essential to the functioning of the professional nurse: altruism, equality, esthetics, freedom, human dignity, justice, and truth.

The *Essentials* document in nursing was preceded by three national studies in 1984 and 1985 recommending improvements in undergraduate education. One of the studies, "To Reclaim a Legacy," the report on humanities in undergraduate education, raises a central question: "Does the curriculum...insure that a graduate with a bachelor's degree will be conversant with the best that has been thought and written about the human condition?" (Bennett, 1984, p. 21). This question is central to the issue of how a liberal education and a professional education both can be achieved in a four-year undergraduate curriculum and is certainly germane to the question of the level at which the first professional degree should be offered.

Sakalys and Watson (1985) reviewed six reports published between 1982 and 1985 that advocated educational reform in the United States. They identified the commonalities in the curriculum recommendations of these reports as being:

1. Restoration of the centrality of the liberal arts in elementary, secondary, postsecondary, and professional education.

2. Increased curricular structure and coherence.

3. Increased emphasis on intellectual skills, such as analytic, problem-solving, and critical thinking skills.

4. Increased emphasis on mastery of basic principles rather than

specific facts.

5. Increased emphasis on fundamental attitudes and values.

6. Increased emphasis on lifelong learning.

7. Decreased specialization at the undergraduate level.

8. Increased emphasis on broad and rigorous baccalaureate education prior to professional education. (Sakalys & Watson, 1985, p. 298)

They concluded that nursing should be restructured so that the first professional degree would be offered at the postbaccalaureate level.

Curtis (1985) offered a proposal for integrating liberal and professional education within the four-year time span, referring to the problem as an "ancient dichotomy." Essentially his proposal called for the faculties in each discipline to examine how their course(s) of study contribute to the knowledge and understanding of the professional students' know-why as opposed to know-how.

Brodie (1986, p. 351) observed in an analysis of the development of American higher education, "Graduate, professional and undergraduate education are inextricably interwoven into the fabric of universities and American life."

The ND Degree

"A nurse is not a 'Medical man.' Nor is she a medical woman" (Woolsey, 1950, Appendix p. 1). Thus spoke Florence Nightingale in 1872 writing to a physician who sought her advice about the training of women as nurses. However, in 1987 a nurse graduate of the ND program at Case Western Reserve University is called a doctor.

The ND program, as conceptualized at Case Western Reserve University, prepares its graduates for clinical practice, clinical scholarship, and a professional career. These goals are reflected in the three-year curriculum. As described by Fitzpatrick (1986), in the first two years students acquire clinical knowledge and skills in preparation for advanced clinical practice in the third year. ND students are enrolled in nursing theory and research courses with MSN students and in professional ethics courses with students in other professions. A concentrated clinical focus from among four areas is selected during the third year and a clinical area of inquiry is undertaken in conjunction with a clinical evaluation project. It should be borne in mind that the ND degree is the first professional degree and thus qualifies the graduate to write the licensure exam.

In the 1985 "Schlotfeldt Lecture" (1986) Schlotfeldt further articulated the need for preparation for professional practice at the postbaccalaureate level. she said that there were "widespread inadequacies in the body of knowledge" currently being taught in baccalaureate nursing programs. She also noted inadequacies in conceptualizations of nursing, in the structure of nursing knowledge, and in the preparation for scholarship. Specifically she cited as problems: (1) having to provide both the liberal and the professional education in a four-year time span; (2) denying nursing's social mission of preserving, restoring, and promoting human health by focusing on the diagnosis and treatment of illness; (3) allowing wide latitude among programs in the development and offering of professional knowledge basic to the practice of nursing; and (4) failing to socialize the student to the role of the scholarly practitioner who seeks answers through systematic inquiry.

The ND program at the Frances Payne Bolton School of Nursing may be viewed as an evolving one with "transition from a very specialized set of graduate level programs to a more integrated approach to the nursing perspective" (Fitzpatrick, 1986, p. 17). The organizing framework for the curriculum includes four focal areas: acute care, long-term care/aging, parent/child/family, and community health/mental health. Future directions for the programs will focus on (1) continued emphasis on clinical scholarship; (2) one-to-one clinical precepting; (3) program flexibility based upon the student's prior learning; (4) renewed emphasis on interdisciplinary learning; and (5) direct and concerted effort toward professional socialization.

According to the 1986–1987 school bulletin (p. 9) the ND graduate is a professional nurse who:

- Is proficient in professional nursing skills.

- Displays interpersonal competence.

- Is able to critically evaluate clinical situations.

- Is ethical in decision making.

- Displays professional values.

- Uses and explicates rationale and data for nursing decisions.

- Critically analyzes nursing phenomena.

- Assumes leadership role in nursing.

- Knows and applies the process of theoretical thinking.

- Uses theoretical and empirical knowledge.

- Uses and tests (knowledge) concepts, models, and theories.

- Assumes responsibility for own learning and professional growth.

- Practices at advanced level in selected focal area.

- Systematically studies a select focal area to advance practice in that area.

- Engages in autonomous, collaborative health care practice.

- Understands information management systems.

- Demonstrates ability to manage health systems and resources.

- Is able to analyze systems to implement change.

- Influences health policy and planning.

The articulation model for the programs offered at the Francis Payne Bolton School of Nursing at Case Western Reserve University are depicted in Figure 1.

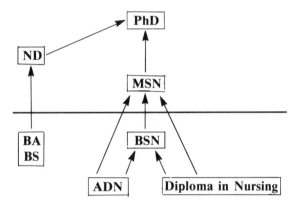

Figure 1. Articulation model at Frances Payne Bolton School of Nursing, Case Western Reserve University. (*Note.* Adapted from Case Western Reserve University *Bulletin, Frances Payne Bolton School of Nursing 1986–87,* p. 8.)

In this configuration the three programs of study are the ND, the MSN, and the PhD (those above the middle line in Figure 1). The ND program offers basic preparation in nursing, the MSN offers specialty preparation, and the PhD offers research preparation. In this model, the ND degree is conceptually on a higher level than the MSN.

At this writing one other institution is planning to implement an ND program (Sakalys & Watson, 1986). The University of Colorado School of Nursing plans to admit the first group of students to the ND program in the fall of 1989 pending university and state approval. The program will be piloted as an advanced honors in health and human caring through the Center for Human Caring, a new initiative in the School. The ND curriculum will include content on human caring; new caring and healing modalities; more use of esthetic means such as music and touch and expressive modes of caring and healing such as journal writing as an expressive mode of self.

The program plans to build upon the experience of Case Western Reserve University and expand the concept of ND by introducing a full health professional nursing model, including advanced practitioner skills, physical as well as psychosocial, while piloting new links between humanities and science through a curriculum focusing on human caring, health and healing. (Watson, 1987, p. 1)

In order to gain acceptance of the new degree program, strategies for internal and external support systems are being implemented. The School is working on piloting new practice roles in traditional and nontraditional settings by working with clinical agencies. Emphasis given to faculty development focuses on new teaching/learning modalities and more self-directed approaches to learning. The third major strategy involves the utilization of state and national advisory committees which act as sounding boards, provide feedback, advise and serve as fund raisers. The committees include representatives from the profession and the community.

Case Western Reserve has been pioneering the ND effort for eight years. More programs are needed so that cross fertilization of ideas can occur, the market place can be tested, faculty can be developed, and public acceptance can be gained.

A number of issues need clarification in regard to the ND program.

1. What is the practice role of the ND graduate? We are accustomed to thinking about the generalist, the specialist, or the doctorally prepared nurse (with the terminal degree). This makes it difficult to fully comprehend the new practice role under the ND degree.

2. Is the ND graduate a beginning or advanced practitioner? The ND graduate at Case Western Reserve is prepared for advanced practice in nursing. In medicine, a new MD graduate is not ready to practice "advanced" medicine. Advance practice comes about after many years of postgraduate training through internships and residencies.

3. How does the ND graduate function differently from the current MSN graduate? Given that the ND graduate is prepared to practice at an advanced level, what is the role of the MSN graduate and do we then need specialty preparation at the master's degree level?

4. What does the job market hold for ND graduates? For what educational and service roles are they prepared? We are accustomed to requiring at least a master's degree in nursing for appointment to a university school of nursing faculty rank. In Illinois a master's degree with a major in nursing is a requirement for state approval of the nursing program leading to licensure as an RN. Will the ND fulfill this requirement? At Case Western Reserve the ND graduate qualifies for appointment to a professorial rank and some graduates have been hired to teach in the ND program (Fitzpatrick, 1986, p. 18). Are they prepared for staff nurse, head nurse, or clinical

specialist roles in the service setting?

5. Should the ND program meet the NLN criteria for the first and the second professional degrees?

6. What organizational structure in the academic unit best accommodates the ND program? Is it necessary to have a model that incorporates faculty responsibility for clinical practice as well as teaching?

7. What are the requirements of faculty in relation to clinical practice?

A longitudinal study is underway at Case Western Reserve and data are being collected on the ND graduates. A preliminary report was issued in 1986 (Fitzpatrick, Boyle, & Anderson). Reporting on 166 graduates through 1986, "Differences in graduate education and employment patterns were noted, with the ND graduates progressing more rapidly and aspiring to more nontraditional roles and higher educational goals" (p. 365).

Recognizing that development of the doctorate as the first professional degree in nursing is a pioneering effort, it will take a number of years and many more programs to resolve these issues or to provide answers. No doubt they will be resolved as the ND program gains in prominence and the value of its graduates becomes known in the health care delivery system.

Three major tasks need to be addressed by programs developing the innovative ND program. These tasks are: (1) developing the practice role, (2) preparing faculty to teach in the program, and (3) gaining public acceptance of the graduates.

THE DOCTORATE AS THE TERMINAL DEGREE

"The exceptional regard that exists for the PhD in academic circles, where presumably most persons know better, has never been fully explained" (Berelson, 1960, pp. 39–40). This observation notwithstanding, the PhD remains the most highly regarded, more revered degree in American higher education.

Two basic models of doctoral degrees as terminal degrees have emerged in nursing. These are the academic degree (the PhD) and the professional degree (the DNS, DSN, or DNSc). Whereas the former degree is awarded by the graduate school, in many instances the latter are awarded by the professional school. These models have derived from the need for doctorally prepared nurses to create the scientific basis for nursing through research and the need for nurses to implement that knowledge in practice.

The PhD is supposed to fulfill the mission of research while the DNS is supposed to fulfill the mission of practice or clinical competence. In reality the distinction between the degrees and among programs is not that clear.

Indeed, Spurr (1970, p. 149) says, "Certainly, the distinction is of limited importance today as the PhD is clearly a professional degree...and we are becoming increasingly aware of the illogicalness of such dichotomies as between pure and applied science or between professional and philosophical studies."

In all but the traditional learned professions of medicine, law, and theology, the professional degree holds lower status and is regarded with less respect than the PhD. Professional degrees awarded by various professions are depicted in Table 1 (Spurr, 1970).

Table 1. Professional Degrees Other Than Nursing.

Profession	Degree
Business Administration	DBA
Dentistry	DDS/DMD
Engineering	DEng
Law	JD
Medicine	MD
Osteopathy	DO
Pharmacy	PharmD
Public Administration	DPA
Public Health	DPH
Social Work	DSW
Theology	DRel/STD
Veterinary Medicine	DVM

In spite of spurts and starts in the development or advancement of doctoral program models, the PhD clearly is in the lead in nursing, and projections indicate that it will remain so. Of the 45 programs awarding doctoral degrees in 1987, 33 programs or 72 percent award the PhD (one program offers both the academic and the professional degree). The distribution of programs appears in Table 2 (National League for Nursing, 1987).

Table 2. Distribution of Doctoral Degrees in Nursing in 1987 (N = 45 Programs)

Degree	Number	Percent
PhD	33	72
DNS	7	17
DNSc	4	8
DSN	1	2
EdD	1	2

There are essentially four educational pathways to the doctorate as the terminal degree for nurses. These are the EdD in nursing (offered only at Teachers College-Columbia University); the PhD or EdD outside of nursing; the PhD in nursing; and the DNS/DSN/DNSc. (Obviously there are many other doctorates available to nurses. The patterns identified here are the most prevalent.)

The first nurse to earn a doctoral degree was Edith Bryan, who was awarded the PhD in psychology and counseling by Johns Hopkins University in 1927 (American Nurses' Foundation, 1969).

Graduations from baccalaureate, master's, and doctoral programs in nursing covering a ten-year span from 1973 through 1982 are shown in Table 3. Among the three programs, doctorate graduations have shown the fastest rate of growth with a 330 percent growth in ten years.

Table 3.   Graduations from Baccalaureate and Higher Degree Programs in Nursing 1973–1982.

Academic Year	Total Number of Graduates	Baccalaureate*	Master's	Doctorate
1982	29033	23855	5039	139
1981	29367	24081	5149	137
1980	29489	24370	4998	121
1979	29874	24994	4755	125
1978	29745	25048	4576	101
1977	28495	24187	4255	53
1976	27311	23452	3800	59
1975	26058	22579	3417	62
1974	22922	20170	2678	74
1973	19627	16957	2624	46

*Does not include RN graduates.
(*Note:* Adapted from National League for Nursing. (1986). *Nursing data review 1985.* New York: Author.)

There were 160 doctorate recipients in nursing in 1984. Of these 7 were male (4 percent) and 153 were female (96 percent); 142 or 92 percent were white, 7 or 4 percent were black, and 6 or 4 percent were other (National Research Council, 1986, pp. 28, 31).

Doctoral programs in nursing by location, focus of study and degree offered are listed in Table 4. It is impossible to differentiate professional from academic degree programs based upon focus of study as reported by the schools.

Table 4. Doctoral Programs in Nursing in 1987.

Location	Focus of Study	Degree
Alabama		
University of Alabama-Birmingham	Clinical Nursing Research Functional Role	DSN
Arizona		
University of Arizona	Clinical Nursing Research	PhD
California		
University of California-San Francisco	Nursing Science Clinical Practice Clinical Research	DNS
	Theory Development Nursing Science Research	PhD
University of California-Los Angeles	Sociocultural Diversity Psycho-physical Environment Health Illness Continuum	DNSc
University of San Diego	Executive Leadership	DNS
Colorado		
University of Colorado	Environmental Health Care Systems Human Care Systems	PhD
District of Columbia		
Catholic University	Nursing Science Clinical Research Related Discipline Professional Role Development	DNSc
Florida		
University of Florida	Clinical Nursing Research	PhD
University of Miami		PhD
Georgia		
Georgia State University	Family and Community Nursing Nursing Education	PhD
Medical College of Georgia	Administration Health Care	PhD

Table 4 continued.

Location	Focus of Study	Degree
Illinois		
Rush University	Clinical Nursing	DNS
University of Illinois	Research	PhD
Indiana		
Indiana University	Administration	DNS
	Clinical Nursing	
Kansas		
University of Kansas	Nursing Research	PhD
Kentucky		
University of Kentucky	Clinical Nursing	PhD
Louisiana		
Louisiana State University	Clinical Nursing	DNS
Maryland		
University of Maryland	Research	PhD
Massachusetts		
Boston College	Clinical Research	PhD
Boston University	Nursing Science	DNS
Michigan		
University of Michigan	Nursing Research	PhD
Wayne State University	Nursing Theory	PhD
	Development	
	Research	
	Practice	
Minnesota		
University of Minnesota	Theory Building	PhD
	Research	
New York		
Adelphia University	Nursing Science	PhD
	Nursing Theory	
	Development	
New York University	Nursing Science	PhD
State University of	Nursing Theory	DNS
New York at Buffalo	Nursing History	
	Research	
Teachers College	Administration	EdD
	Professional Role	
University of Rochester	Clinical Research	PhD
	Theory Building	

Table 4 continued.

Location	Focus of Study	Degree
Ohio		
Case Western Reserve University	Nursing Science Research	PhD
Ohio State University	Nursing Science	PhD
Oregon		
Oregon Health Sciences University	Theory Building Research	PhD
Pennsylvania		
University of Pennsylvania	Clinical Investigation Administration Teaching	PhD
University of Pittsburgh	Research	PhD
Widener University	Education	DNSc
Rhode Island		
University of Rhode Island	Clinical Nursing Research	PhD
South Carolina		
University of South Carolina	Nursing Theory Nursing Research	PhD
Texas		
Texas Woman's University	Theory Development Clinical Research	PhD
University of Texas-Austin	Clinical Nursing Research Administration	PhD
Utah		
University of Utah	Nursing Research Clinical Nursing	PhD
Virginia		
George Mason University	Administration	DNSc
Medical College of Virginia/Virginia Commonwealth University	Administration Clinical Science (a joint program with microbiology immunology)	PhD
University of Virginia	Psychosocial Nursing Complex Organization	PhD

Table 4 continued.

Location	Focus of Study	Degree
Washington		
University of Washington	Nursing Science	PhD
Wisconsin		
University of Wisconsin-Madison	Nursing and Psychology	PhD
University of Wisconsin-Milwaukee	Nursing Research	PhD

(*Note:* Adapted from National League for Nursing. (1987). *Doctoral Programs in Nursing.* New York: Author).

Professional versus Academic Degrees

Addressing the Association of American Universities in 1906, President David Starr Jordan of Stanford observed that "not all who talk of research, even in Germany, shall enter the kingdom" (National Research Council, 1969, p. 9).

This position is supported by the findings of Pitel and Vian (1975) who reported in their survey of nurses doctorally prepared that 3.5 percent were engaged in research as their primary position and research was considered to be a major responsibility of the primary position by 31.5 percent of the respondents. In a later study reported in 1983 it was found that "...few nurses are employed primarily for conduct of research and, in the aggregate, an average of only 12 percent of work time is reportedly focused on research activities..." (Brimmer, Skoner, Pender, Williams, Fleming, & Werley, p. 164).

These findings would seem to refute the position that the PhD socializes one into the research role and the case for the academic degree over the professional degree as a basis for research productivity.

The Council of Graduate Schools in their joint statement with the Association of Graduate Schools (1966) differentiated between the professional and the academic degree as follows:

> The professional Doctor's degree should be the highest university award given in a particular field in recognition of completion of academic *preparation for professional practice,* whereas the Doctor of Philosophy degree should be given in recognition of *preparation for research* whether the particular field of learning is pure or applied. (p. 3)

The professional doctorate also carries with it the obligation to give service to the public in the chosen field (Council of Graduate Schools, 1966).

At least one other profession is also debating the issue of academic versus professional preparation. In psychology the research-oriented scientist and the clinically oriented practitioner traditionally have been educated in the same graduate program (Staff, 1987). In recent years a number of proprietary programs have evolved offering specialty training for practitioners and awarding a PsyD degree. The concern over quality has given rise to a push for a common core curriculum for all psychology programs. The American Psychological Association at a recent conference voted for diversity while calling for research and scientific inquiry to be an essential part of all training programs and asking the accrediting body to develop criteria which reflect differential foci.

Lancaster (1982) studies the 21 doctoral programs in nursing listed in the 1980–81 NLN doctoral program listing. He found no significant differences between the 14 PhD and the 7 DNS programs in curricula designs; nor was the dissertation research well differentiated and statements of philosophy and objectives "did not clearly differentiate the purpose and outcomes of the two types of doctoral programs" (p. 65).

Regarding the question of which doctoral model to follow, a number of opinions prevail in nursing.

> Cleland (1978) indicated her preference for the professional doctorate. I personally favor the...professional doctorate. It will be essential for the recognition of nursing's role in patient care management in the health service setting. We must be clear, however, about our expectations and goals. The professional doctorate is designed to prepare a utilizer of research rather than an investigator, and its primary focus should be upon expert clinical practice. (p. 632)

Lash (1987) challenges long-held assumptions that the PhD program cannot accommodate the practice component of nursing, citing engineering and psychology as two practice fields utilizing the PhD. She cites this fact and nursing's failure to develop unique non-PhD practice-oriented curricula as reasons:

> ...for nursing to modify the PhD model in ways to improve the fit between the goals of nursing and the degree, rather than to continue to experiment with the professional model that has not produced the intended results and does not have the same social utility/acceptability as the PhD (p. 100)

Hechenberger (1983) believes that the "two major types of doctoral degrees in nursing...should continue... Doctoral nursing programs should begin to look less alike and become reflective of the strengths of a given school" (p. 183). Moreover, she says programs will specialize and will recruit and attract students whose interests are congruent with faculty expertise.

In 1982, Grace held the view that:

...the time is now for the consideration of the need for a parallel professional doctoral pattern that is designed to prepare the expert practitioner and teacher of nursing. This pattern is necessary if we are to bring research findings into the practice of nursing, thereby changing care delivery. (p. 14)

Andreoli (1987) contends that nursing clinical specialization should be at the doctoral level and that the degree offered should be the DSN, the doctor of science in nursing. She argues that the DSN: (1) flows logically from the MSN which would be the first professional degree preparing a generalist, (2) correctly identifies nursing as the major rather than science, and (3) will clearly identify the profession to the public. She proposes that nurses who want to do research obtain a PhD. Using her model, the career path would be MSN to DSN to PhD.

Forni and Welch (1987) propose two higher education models called the academic model and the professional model. The believe that the model nursing chooses to follow in higher education will directly influence the development of doctoral programs in nursing. In their conceptualization nursing would follow the academic model to the doctorate leading to the PhD and there would be no practice degree at the doctorate level. Clinical specialization would remain at the master's degree level and the doctorate as the terminal degree would be reserved for the pursuit of scholarship and knowledge development through research and theory building/testing (Forni and Welch, 1987). Two educational pathways to clinical specialization and/or research are shown in Figure 2. This model, in some respects, more closely resembles that followed in other professional disciplines (dentistry and medicine) in that the master's degree follows the basic preparatory program in the discipline (either post-BSN or post-ND).

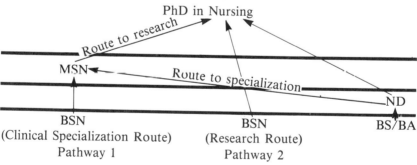

Figure 2. Two proposed educational pathways to clinical specialization and/or research. [*Note:* Ferni, P., & Welch, M. 1987. The professional versus the academic model: A dilemma for nursing. *Journal of Professional Nursing, 3* (5).]

Donaldson and Crowley (1978) writing about the relationship of the discipline to practice explain it this way:

Although the discipline and the profession are inextricably linked and greatly influence each other's substance, they must be distinguished from each other. Failure to recognize the existence of the discipline as a body of knowledge that is separate from the activities of practitioners has contributed to the fact that nursing has been viewed as a vocation rather than a profession. ...Since the university traditionally has been the locus of development of theoretical knowledge, the professional disciplines were eventually housed there along with the academic disciplines. The location of professional disciplines such as nursing in institutions such as universities, which are primarily concerned with human knowledge as a product rather than service, does not change the accountability of these disciplines for societal needs and the practical aim of their associated professions. (p. 117)

CURRENT ISSUES AND FUTURE TRENDS

There is now strong support among nursing leaders for doctoral education in nursing. When the Institute of Medicine (IOM) report was published in 1983 there was one recommendation which called for the federal government to provide financial support to increase the supply of nurses with master's and doctoral degrees "in nursing and relevant disciplines" (IOM, 1983, p. 151). This reference to relevant disciplines was rebutted by Ruby Wilson and Dorothy Novello, members of the study Committee on Nursing and Nursing Education. In doing so they said:

> The development of knowledge and competencies unique to nursing must be produced by nurses with advanced education in nursing and whose research is focused on clinical nursing practice... This expectation is not different from that in other disiciplines where advanced degrees or academic study are offered...(IOM, p. 152).

Brown (1985, p. 12) predicted a glut of doctorally prepared nurses by 1997. I do not believe this will be the case. Given the slow rate of output of doctorates in nursing and the pressing needs for faculty with doctoral preparation in university nursing programs and for leadership positions I believe it will be many years before we meet initial market demands. Brimmer, Skoner, Pender, Williams, Fleming, and Werley (1983) support this view, predicting that by the end of the 1980s only two-thirds of nurses with doctorates who are active in the workforce will be under 65 years of age. Moreover, Anderson, Roth, and Palmer (1985) reported that their survey data indicated that fewer than 25 percent of nursing faculty in baccalaureate and higher degree programs hold earned doctorates. AACN (1987) data for 1986–1987 show that 31.8 percent of the faculty from reporting schools hold doctorates (p. 7).

In nursing we offer the first professional degree (usually the BSN, but also the MN or MSN, and the ND); the second professional degree (the MSN); and now a third professional degree (the DSN/DNS/DNSc). In medicine there is only one professional degree, the MD, and advanced education may be attained in related fields leading to the PhD, MPH or the like. In dentistry there also is one professional degree (DDS or DMD) with graduate degrees for advanced specialty practice in dentistry leading to the master's degree (awarded postdoctorally).

All this makes for a fuzzy picture when attempting to arrive at a model for nursing that is at once consonant with the needs of society, with the goals of the profession, and with the mission of the university, while paralleling other professional disciplines of high stature.

The MD degree is and has always been the "practice" degree in medicine. The medical profession has been concerned with high levels of clinical competence since the turn of the century at least. Competence in caring for patients through research and clinical practice is achieved in incremental stages of noncredit, postgraduate, postdoctoral fellowships. In 1920 only six states required a medical internship, but by 1930 practically all graduates served an internship whether or not it was required (National Research Council, 1969, p. 11). The American Opthamological Society offered the first specialty board examination in 1916 and others followed in time. Fellowships were awarded for advanced study in basic sciences and research and were usually tied to a university rather than a hospital.

Nursing has no parallel in clinical practice in terms of service appointments following the basic preparatory program. The master's degree is said to prepare for specialty or advanced practice. What role then does the professional doctorate serve in this scenario? I can only say that nursing would do well to emphasize clinical expertise through the higher levels as does medicine.

It is interesting to note that the University of Minnesota in 1914 initiated graduate degrees (post-MD) in medicine, either the master's degree or PhD. The following year the program of study was extended to the Mayo Foundation in Rochester. The program attracted many "fellows" through the 1930s but the movement was not taken up by other universities and other means of postgraduate education were devised by the various specialty societies in order to meet this recognized need for practical and research training beyond the basic preparatory program (National Research Council, 1969, pp. 12–13).

In light of this discussion, what does the future hold for doctoral education in nursing? These are my predictions:

1. Doctoral programs in nursing will continue to be developed at a rapid rate until market needs are met.

2. There will continue to be at least two educational pathways to the doctorate as the terminal degree: the academic and professional doctorates.

3. The debate will continue over which degree best serves nursing,

the professional or the academic degree.

4. A doctorate in nursing will be the preferred degree among degree alternatives.

5. Doctoral education for nurses in other disciplines will continue to be a viable alternative but will carry very limited import among nursing faculty

6. University nursing faculty will be required to have the doctoral degree for appointment to a professorial rank.

7. The Doctor of Nursing (ND) degree will gain in acceptance and more programs will be developed; this will further clarify the distinctions between technical and professional nursing at the entry level.

8. As more nurses with doctorates in nursing assume faculty positions we will increasingly see the nature and dimensions of doctoral program models expand and be derived from a stronger nursing base.

9. The job market for nurses with doctorates in nursing will expand beyond educational settings.

Some of the remaining issues to be addressed associated with doctoral program development are:

1. Impact on other nursing programs in the academic unit especially the undergraduate program.

2. Need for restructuring the master's degree program.

3. Changes in the expectations of faculty for appointment to rank and in their job responsibilities.

4. Impact of doctorally prepared nurses on health care delivery costs and quality.

5. Need to monitor quality of programs.

Nursing also faces a number of challenges for: (1) meeting the university expectations for teaching, research, and service; and (2) fulfilling the practice role of the profession. The question remains: How can the scholarly and research requirements for disciplinary status be reconciled with the service requirements of the profession?

In speaking about doctoral program developments Norrris (1985) predicts that, "administrative and senior faculty leadership that moves nursing faculty into meeting the same academic standards as faculty in other disciplines will be aggressive. More than any other change in schools initiating a doctoral program, this process is critical" (p. 12).

In consideration of these dual challenges it would seem that a major task confronting nursing leaders and university faculty is to develop doctoral programs in nursing that will produce nurses in sufficient numbers and kind to fulfill their requisite roles: that of researcher who will contribute to nursing's body of knowledge and that of practitioner who will translate the research findings into the practice of nursing.

It further would seem apparent that two routes to doctoral education for nurses, namely the academic and the professional degrees, could accomplish this task. Yet, we have observed that the PhD, the academic or research degree, is gaining in popularity among nursing doctoral programs. We have also observed that there is little difference between the two degrees in relation to the curricula or career paths of their graduates. We have further observed that few nurses with doctorates are engaged in research. Moreover we have heard that the PhD is an appropriate framework within which to offer the practice component.

What can we conclude from all this? Given the pluralistic nature of our society and of our educational network, it seems apparent that a multiplicity of programs will continue to exist and thrive. This phenomenon will serve to enrich the educational experience of the graduates and enhance the opportunities for doctoral study in nursing. What seems apparent is that there is no perfect program for preparing nurses to become researchers, teachers, administrators, and practitioners. Perhaps we should heed Matarazzo (1971, p. 63) who observed that, "...it is probably the personal characteristics of the man (or woman), and not his academic degree per se which will help determine his degree of contribution to our vast, ever-increasing output of new scientific knowledge." Be that as it may, nursing will continue, for some time into the future, to strive for (and to agonize over) its rightful place in the academic community. We have yet to fully overcome our early heritage as handmaiden to the physician and the gender burdens (lack of equality and worth) attendant to a predominately female profession. Given these caveats it seems prudent that we are taking stock of where we have been, where we are at the present, and where we are going in the area of doctoral education of nurses. Whatever model we choose we must pursue it with excellence as both our individual and collective goal.

REFERENCES

American Association of Colleges of Nursing. (1986). *Essentials of college and university education for professional nursing: Final report.* Washington, DC: Author.

American Association of Colleges of Nursing. (1987). *Report on nursing faculty salaries 1986–87.* Washington, DC: Author.

American Nurses' Foundation, Inc. (1969). Directory of nurses with earned doctoral degrees. *Nursing Research, 18* (5), 465–480.

Anderson, E., Roth, P., & Palmer, I. S. (1985). A national survey of the need for doctorally prepared nurses in academic settings and health service agencies. *Journal of Professional Nursing, 1* (1), 23–33.

Andreoli, K. G. (1987). Specialization and graduate curricula: Finding the fit. *Nursing and Health Care, 8* (2), 65–69.

Bennett, W. J. (1984, November 28). To reclaim a legacy: Text of report on humanities in education. *Chronicle of Higher Education,* pp. 16–21.

Berelson, B. (1960). *Graduate Education in the United States.* New York: McGraw-Hill.

Brimmer, P. F., Skoner, M. M., Pender, N. J., Williams, C. G., Fleming, J. W. & Werley, H. H. (1983). Nurses with doctoral degrees: Education and employment characteristics. *Research in Nursing and Health, 6,* 157–165.

Brodie, B. (1986). Impact of doctoral programs on nursing education. *Journal of Professional Nursing, 2* (6), 350–357.

Brown, B. J. (1985, July). *Diversity of doctoral education.* Paper presented at the American Association of Colleges of Nursing Deans' Summer Seminar, Aspen, CO.

Brubacher, J. S. (1962). The evolution of professional education. In N. B. Henry (Ed.), *Education for the professions* (pp. 47–67). Chicago: University of Chicago.

Case Western Reserve University. (1986, September). *Frances Payne Bolton School of Nursing Bulletin 1986-87. 10* (4).

Cleland, V. (1976). Developing a doctoral program. *Nursing Outlook, 24* (10), 631–635.

Council of Graduate Schools in the United States. (1966). *The doctor's degree in professional fields.* A statement by the Association of Graduate Schools and the Council of Graduate Schools in the United States. Washington, DC: Author.

Curtis, M. H. (1985). Confronting an ancient dichotomy: A proposal for integrating liberal and professional education. *Phi Kappa Phi Journal, 65* (3), 10–12.

Donaldson, S. K., & Crowley, D. M. (1978). The discipline of nursing. *Nursing Outlook, 26* (2), 113–120.

Eells, W. C., & Haswell, H. A. (1960). *Academic degrees.* Washington, DC: U.S. Government Printing Office.

Fitzpatrick, J. J. (1986). *The N.D. program: Integration of past and future,* The Schlotfeldt Lecture. Cleveland: Case Western Reserve University.

Fitzpatrick, J. J., Boyle, K. K. & Anderson, R. M. (1986). Evaluation of the doctor of nursing (ND) program: Preliminary findings. *Journal of Professional Nursing, 2* (6), 365–372.

Flexner, A. (1930). *Universities: American English German.* New York: Oxford University Press.

Forni, P., & Welch, M. (1987). The professional versus the academic model:

A dilemma for nursing education. *Journal of Professional Nursing, 3* (5).

Grace, H. (1978). The development of doctoral education in nursing: In historical perspective. *Journal of Nursing Education, 17* (4), 17–27.

Grace, H. K. (1982). Building nursing knowledge: The current state of doctoral education in nursing. In J. J. Fitzpatrick (Compiler). *Proceedings of the Sixth National Forum on Doctoral Education in Nursing* (pp. 1–14). Cleveland: Case Western Reserve University School of Nursing.

Grace, H. K. (1983). Doctoral education in nursing: Dilemmas and directions. In Norma Chaska (Ed.), *The nursing profession: A time to speak* (pp. 146–155). New York: McGraw-Hill.

Hechenberger, N. B. (1983). The future in master's and doctoral education in nursing. In *Perspectives in nursing 1983–85* (pp. 179–185). New York: National League for Nursing.

Institute of Medicine. (1983). *Nursing and nursing education: Public policies and private actions.* Washington, DC: National Academy Press.

Lancaster, L. E. (1982). A comparison and development of models for the doctor of philosophy in nursing and the doctor of nursing science degrees (Doctoral dissertation, Vanderbilt University, 1982). *University Microfilms International.*

Lash, A. A. (1987). The nature of the doctor of philosphy degree: Evolving conceptions. *Journal of Professional Nursing, 3* (2), 92–101.

Matarazzo, J. D. (1971). Perspective. In *Future directions of doctoral education for nurses* (DHEW Publication No. NIH 72–82, pp. 50–105). Washington, DC: U.S. Government Printing Office.

Matarazzo, J. D., & Abdellah, F. G. (1971). Doctoral education for nurses in the United States. *Nursing Research, 20* (5), 404–414.

Murphy, J. F. (1981). Doctoral education in, of, and for nursing: An historical analysis. *Nursing Outlook, 29* (11), 645–649.

National League for Nursing. (1986). *Nursing Data Review 1985.* New York: Author.

National League for Nursing. (1987). *Doctoral programs in nursing 1986–87.* New York: Author.

National Research Council. (1969). *The invisible university.* Washington, DC: National Academy of Sciences.

National Research Council. (1978). *A century of doctorates.* Washington, DC: National Academy of Sciences.

National Research Council. (1986). *Summary report 1984. Doctorate recipients from United States universities.* Washington, DC: National Academy Press.

Newman, J. H. (1976). *The idea of a university.* London: Oxford University Press.

Newman, M. A. (1975). The professional doctorate in nursing: A position paper. *Nursing Outlook, 23* (11), 704–706.

Norris, C. M. (1985). The PhD in nursing programs: A five-year projection.

Nurse Educator, 10 (2), 6–11.

Peplau, H. E. (1966). Nursing's two routes to doctoral degrees. *Nursing Forum, V* (2), 57–67.

Pitel, M. & Vian, J. (1975). Analysis of nurse-doctorates. *Nursing Research, 24* (5), 340–351.

Rashdall, H. (1936). *The universities of Europe in the middle ages. Vol. I.* London: Oxford University Press.

Rogers, M. E. (1966). Doctoral education in nursing. *Nursing Forum, V* (2), 75–82.

Sakalys, J. A., & Watson, J. W. (1985). New directions in higher education; A review of trends. *Journal of Professional Nursing, 1* (5), 293–299.

Sakalys, J. A., & Watson, J. W. (1986). Professional education: Post-baccalaureate education for professional nursing. *Journal of Professional Nursing, 2* (2), 91–97.

Schlotfeldt, R. M. (1966). Doctoral study in basic disciplines—A choice for nurses. *Nursing Forum, V* (2), 68–74.

Schlotfeldt, R. M. (1978). The professional doctorate: Rationale and characteristics. *Nursing Outlook, 26* (5), 302–311.

Spurr, S. H. (1970). *Academic degree structures: Innovative approaches.* New York: McGraw-Hill.

Staff. (1987, July 1). Psychologists say graduate schools shouldn't impose single standard. *Chronicle of Higher Education,* p. 12.

Stevenson, J. S., & Woods, N. F. (1986). Nursing science and contemporary science: Emerging paradigms. In G. E. Sorensen (Ed.), *Setting the agenda for the year 2000: Knowledge development in nursing* (pp. 6–20). Kansas City, MO: American Academy of Nursing.

Tschudin, M. S. (1966). Doctoral preparation in other disciplines. *Nursing Forum, V* (2), 51–56.

Watson, J. (1987). *Postbaccalaureate model development.* Unpublished paper, University of Colorado, School of Nursing, Denver.

Woolsey, A. H. (1950). *A century of nursing.* New York: Putnam.

6 SPECIALIZED ACCREDITATION OF DOCTORAL PROGRAMS IN NURSING: TO BE OR NOT TO BE

Jeannette R. Spero, PhD, RN, FAPHA

INTRODUCTION

It's time for completion of the accreditation self-study report! The faculty and administrators are worried and under stress. New committees have been created requiring additional time and effort on the part of faculty, students, and staff. The day-to-day activities essential to the operation of the educational unit continue but, during this special period, priority is given to the collection and analysis of data necessary for completing the necessary report. There is a wild flurry of last-minute corrections and much retyping. New tables are added and old tables are revised. At last, the report is bound and sent on its way. Everyone breathes a collective sigh of relief, and life in the educational unit soon returns to normal.

Anxieties peak once again at the time of the site visit. For several weeks immediately following the site visit, there is much preoccupation with the site visitors' report and the conduct of the visit. There are cyclical periods of elation and depression among faculty, students, and staff dependent upon one's perception of the events. Finally, a feeling of acceptance and, yes, resignation prevails because the site visitors made it very clear to all that the final determination of the educational program's accreditation status will be made by the review board of the accrediting association (Lewis, 1983).

Why, one must wonder, do educators willingly submit to the intellectual and emotional pressures associated with accreditation? What factors contributed to the development of a voluntary system of accreditation for postsecondary education in the United States? What is the difference be-

75

tween general/institutional accreditation and specialized/programmatic accreditation? What are the stated purposes and perceived values of the accreditation process? Has a relationship between accreditation and quality of graduate education been established?

This chapter will address all of the above questions in summary form because each is relevant to the question that has been posed regarding the need for specialized accreditation of doctoral programs in nursing. The chapter will conclude with the findings of an opinion survey of deans or their designees currently offering doctoral programs in nursing.

DEVELOPMENT OF VOLUNTARY ACCREDITATION OF POSTSECONDARY EDUCATION IN THE UNITED STATES

The voluntary system of educational accreditation currently extant is strictly an American phenomenon. No other country has a voluntary, non-governmental process for evaluating its educational institutions. In the United States, "...the primary responsibility for education rests, not with the federal government, not with peer group agencies, but with the states and local governments" (Millard, 1979, p. 121). During the early developlment of institutions of higher education, most states, with the exception of New York, tended to adopt a somewhat laissez-faire attitude toward the regulation of higher education (Brubacher & Rudy, 1976). In 1787, the University of the State (the New York Board of Regents) was required by law to annually review every college in the state; to register each curriculum at each institution and report the results to the legislature. Shortly thereafter, other states adopted similar legislation. Thus, accreditation began at the state level (Harcleroad, 1980).

In 1867, the United States Bureau of Education was established and had as one of its tasks a listing of all collegiate institutions. It defined a collegiate institution as one "...authorized to give degrees and which reported college students in attendance" (Semrow, 1982, p. 384). This definition was revised in 1965 by the Carnegie Foundation for the Advancement of Teaching to read, "a collegiate institution was one which possessed no less than $200,000 of productive endowment, had at least six chairs of instruction and required four years of college preparation for admission and 120 semester hours for graduation" (Semrow, 1982, p. 384).

By 1895 four regional associations—New England, Middle States, Southern, and North Central—had been established by educators to alleviate continuing problems in higher education related to the development of new academic disciplines, diversity of institutions, and the breakdown of the classical curriculum. It was not, however, until 1912 that the North Central Association established specific criteria for accreditation and subsequently published the first list of fully accredited institutions. Prior to the establishment of the early regional associations, the American Medical Association became, in 1847, the first health-related association to engage in voluntary programmatic accreditation thereby establishing the viability of specialized accrediting organizations (Harcleroad, 1980).

Accrediting associations continued to proliferate during the nineteenth and twentieth centuries. Established associations revised criteria and modified review procedures in response to criticism from the higher education community. The 1950s and 1960s was a period of vast change which profoundly affected postsecondary education and the accrediting process. One major factor was the massive increases in federal funds available to institutions and students following World War II. In 1968, the Division of Accreditation and Institutional Eligibility was established in the United States Office of Education to determine institutional eligibility for federal funds. In its determination of "eligibility," the United States Office of Education relied upon the listing of accredited institutions provided by officially recognized accrediting associations (Trivett, 1976). The Education Amendments of 1972 expanded the definition of postsecondary institutions to include all forms of education beyond high school. This led to a precipitous increase in the number of educational programs eligible for federal funds and placed serious demands upon accrediting bodies. The proliferation of postsecondary institutions led to abuses on the part of some institutions, and the public demanded consumer protection by holding accrediting associations accountable for their accrediting actions.

Voluntary accreditation in nursing developed for many of the same reasons that accreditation developed in other health-related disciplines and in higher education. In the late nineteenth century there was much concern expressed by representatives of the profession about the quality of and standards for nursing education. It was not, however, until the 1920s that the National Organization for Public Health Nursing accredited "advanced programs in public health nursing." IN 1939, the National League for Nursing Education provided accrediting services to both collegiate and hospital programs. Other nursing and health-related associations continued to engage in independent accreditation activities until in 1949 a unified accrediting service for nursing education, the National Nursing Accrediting Service (NNAS), was established under the aegis of six national nursing organizations. In 1952, the activities of NNAS were transferred to the Division of Education of the National League for Nursing (National League for Nursing [NLN], 1964).

Since assuming responsibility for the accreditation of nursing education programs, the NLN has conducted several accreditation studies, the most recent of which was completed in 1981. In reviewing the draft of the NLN Accreditation Study Final Report, Shannon (1981) addressed satisfactions and dissatisfactions with the accreditation process as revealed in the study, many of which are similar to criticism cited in this chapter's section on the purposes, uses, process, and criticisms of accreditation.

In 1975 the Council on Postsecondary Accreditation (COPA) was formed in an effort to unify all voluntary accrediting activities and "to interrelate (1) the general public, (2) users of accreditation, (3) general accrediting agencies, (4) specialized accrediting agencies, and (5) national associations representing institutions" (COPA, 1979, pp. 2–3). The Council on Postsecondary Accreditation has undertaken several studies on various aspects of the accreditation process and continues to study problems related to self-study procedures and standards, institutional site visitations, the peer review process, and the evaluation of eduational quality (Harcleroad, 1980).

TYPES OF ACCREDITATION

There are two types of accreditation: (1) general, which deals with an institution in its totality; and (2) specialized, which focuses on special programs or fields within single disciplines (Semrow, 1982). General or institutional accreditation is conducted by the regional accrediting associations. In addition to examination of the institution's educational programs, regional accreditation includes assessment of other areas such as student personnel and support services, finances, and administrative organization and support (Millard, 1983). Successful accreditation of this type represents an expression of confidence on the part of the accrediting agency in the institution's mission, purposes, resources, present performance, and long-range ability to maintain and enhance its performance (Dressel, 1978).

Specialized accreditation is conducted by accrediting associations representing specific professional, occupational, or disciplinary areas. The primary purpose of specialized accreditation is to assure that the purposes and accomplishments of practice-oriented programs meet societal needs for appropriately qualified professionals. Accreditation of specialized programs usually requires that the practice-oriented program be housed in an institution that has received general accreditation. Thus in specialized accreditation, a specific program is reviewed in depth and, to some extent, also is reviewed within the context of the total institution. The degree to which the total institution is examined during the conduct of specialized accreditation varies among accrediting associations.

Programmatic or specialized accreditation applies to specific programs at baccalaureate or postbaccalaureate levels. "General accreditation, in contrast, involves a composite judgment on an entire institution, and such program distinctions as are made are usually by degree or level rather than by specific program" (Dressel, 1978, p. 2).

ACCREDITATION: PURPOSES, USES, PROCESS, AND CRITICISMS

There are many definitions of accreditation, the majority of which denote a relationship between accreditation and institutional quality. The Council of Graduate Schools in the United States (1978) defined accreditation in postsecondary education as ". . . voluntary, non-governmental, self-regulatory process—the granting of which signifies that an institution or program meets or exceeds a level of quality considered to be necessary for that particular institution or program to achieve its stated purposes and thereby meet its responsibilities to all of its publics" (p. 8).

Harcleroad and Dickey (1975) stated that accreditation serves as "the major factor in quality control for our institutions of higher education and for various professional and specialized programs" (p. 7). The North Central Association defines accreditation as a ". . . non-governmental, voluntary means of attesting to the quality of educational institutions and of assisting institutions to improve their programs" (Manning, 1982, p. 63).

The National League for Nursing (1985) states that the purposes of accreditation of programs in nursing are:

1. To foster the continuous development and improvement in quality of educational programs throughout the United States and its territories.

2. To evaluate nursing programs in relation both to their stated purposes and objectives and to the established criteria for accreditation.

3. To involve administrators of the governing institutions and the administrators, faculties, and students of nursing programs in the process of continuous self-study and improvement of their programs.

4. To bring together practitioners, administrators, faculty, and students in an activity directed toward improving educational preparation for nursing practice.

5. To provide an external peer-review process (p. 3).

The uses of accreditation are variously identified as: (1) certifying to the public that an institution has met established standards; (2) assisting institutions in determining the acceptability of transfer credits; (3) involving faculty and staff in institutional evaluation and planning; (4) establishing standards of professional certification and thereby providing assistance to prospective employers in identifying qualified personnel; and (5) providing one of several considerations to be used as a basis for determining eligibility for federal funds (McCloskey, 1984; U.S. Department of Health, Education and Welfare, 1980). The ultimate value of accreditation is related to the assumption, on the part of the public, that "accredited" means "legitimate" and, therefore, accredited institutions and programs are bonafide providers of educational services worthy of the government's investment of funds and worthy of a student's investment of time, effort, and money (Levin, 1981).

To the uninitiated, the process of accreditation seems very simple and straightforward: (1) identify those factors that are essential to a functionally effective educational unit; (2) establish criteria and standards which reflect those factors; and (3) encourage institutions by means of a formalized review process to demonstrate that the essential factors are operationalized (Astin, 1980). The factors generally considered in an accreditation review are administration and governance, finances and budget, faculty, students, curriculum, and resources. These factors are further elaborated by the establishment of subsets within each category and by stating components in the form of criteria. The educational unit being reviewed is expected to describe the ways in which criteria are met and to provide substantiating qualitative and quantitative data in the form of a self-study report. The self-study report is reviewed by a volunteer visiting team, either selected or elected by representatives of the accrediting association to make a site visit. Following the site visit, both the visitors' report and the self-study report are reviewed by the accrediting board of the association, although this step in the process may vary in keeping with procedures established by individual accrediting associations.

Since its inception, accreditation has been a target for both bouquets and barbs. Petersen (1978) declared that many of the faults ascribed to the accreditation process are based more on "personal biases, isolated incidents, or rumors on what has happened" (p. 305) than on an objective assessment of events. Supporters of the process assert that: (1) it provides an external stimulus for the improvement of educational programs and prevents academic stagnation (Reinert, 1949); (2) it encourages objective self-evaluation, identification of deficits, and the development of plans to correct the deficits thus ensuring increased quality of the educational program (Young, Chambers, Kells, and Associates, 1983); and (3) evaluation be peers who have participated in the establishment of criteria and procedures adds validity to the process (Newton, 1966). Young, et al. (1983), asserted that "the genius of accreditation is that it began with the impossible task of defining educational quality and in just twenty-five years evolved, by trial and error, into a process that advances educational quality" (p. 13).

The gainsayers assert that: (1) the criteria, even with descriptors, are insufficient to measure program quality (Demaree, 1980; Troutt, 1981); (2) there are "hidden standards" behind the criteria (Petersen, 1978); and (3) the accreditation process emphasizes form over substance "assuming that outcomes not easily measured by direct assessment are largely a result of good facilities, good faculty and selectivity in admissions" (Dressel, 1978, p. 12). Accreditation has been described as a self-serving process conducted by "a series of mutual protection societies designed to inhibit innovation, restrict trade or protect institutions or programs from public accountability" (Millard, 1983, p. 34). One could add to the above criticism Semrow's (1977) contention that self-studies that are evaluative in nature are "the exception rather than the rule" (p. 84). He argues that if the self-study serves as the basis for review, then to point out problems which might otherwise be overlooked, is an invitation to denial of accreditation.

One of the earliest and most quoted critics of accreditation was Samuel P. Capen, Chancellor of the University of Buffalo, who, in a speech, referred to the accrediting associations as the seven devils and stated,

> "Responsible administrators of influential institutions...are tired of having the educational and financial policies of their institutions dictated by a horde of irresponsible outsiders, each representing a separate, selfish interest." (cited in Young, et. al., 1983, p. 13)

In his speech, Capen challenged the leaders of the universities to unite in the decision that the agencies 'shall live no longer.' Obviously, Capen's hope that the accrediting associations would meet their demise has not seen fruition. Voluntary accreditation, despite the controversy which surrounds it, has established its place in American society.

The accrediting associations have responded to criticisms by studying various components of the process. Criteria have been revised and procedures modified. In some associations, board members and site visitors are no longer appointed but are now drawn from a list of volunteers elected by the membership. Consumers have been added to boards, and the administrative head of the educational unit being reviewed is invited to attend the final review and respond to reviewers' comments for the purpose of clarification. In speaking of the many changes in the National League for Nursing accrediting process, Hart (1984) stated,

> ...as important or significant as these changes might be, the fact remains that programs will achieve and retain accreditation if they have a sufficient number of qualified faculty, adequate financial resources, a soundly conceived, well organized and logically developed curriculum that focuses on the knowledge and practice of nursing, a comprehensive evaluation plan that is operational and a critical mass of qualified students. This is how it has always been, that is probably how it will always be and how it should be, or, to put it another way, while many changes have been made, nothing of consequence has really changed at all. (p. 19)

ACCREDITATION AND GRADUATE EDUCATION

Although the effectiveness of accreditation generally has been recognized by the higher education community, accreditation of graduate education in particular has posed a variety of thought-provoking questions. Issues not yet satisfactorily resolved in accreditation of graduate education relate to: (1) who shall accredit? (2) for what purpose? (3) at what levels? (4) in what fields?, and (5) according to what procedures? (Council of Graduate Schools in the United States, 1978).

The maintenance and improvement of program quality always has been a dominant concern in graduate education. Anderson (1978) observes that while "higher education could tolerate wide diversity and lesser quality in undergraduate programs, and even at the master's level. . .it registers deep concern when the quality of the doctorate is diluted" (p. 279). The higher education community has come to expect that any university of stature involved in graduate work and research will engage in recurrent reviews directed by the graduate dean and graduate faculty.

Doctoral programs are generally of two types: (1) the research-oriented degree program directed toward scholarship and the acquisition of new knowledge and (2) the practice-oriented degree program which has as its basic focus the application or transmission of existing knowledge (Dressel, 1978). Graduate education implies advanced, intensive, and purposeful study that builds upon the knowledge base and intellectual maturity of students. There is great diversity among graduate programs. Some are fully prescribed; others, although prescribed, may contain some elements of flexibility; and still others may be highly individualized (Dressel, 1978). This diversity makes it difficult to evaluate doctoral education by means of the traditional form and structure indices used in the accreditation process. Lawrence and Green (1980) believe that accreditation may actually impede assessment of institutional or program quality. They note that whereas the accrediting community asserts a relationship between quality and accreditation, it has not fared well in its attempts to define the actual attributes of institutional or programmatic quality. Whereas there is general consensus that quality is an elusive concept (Griffiths, 1978; Lawrence & Green, 1980; Scott, 1981), there is also general agreement that "when an institution's mission is well established and understood, it creates a frame of reference for assessing program quality" (Caruthers, 1980, p. 83).

Griffiths (1978) contended that accreditation of doctoral programs is not sufficient to ensure their excellence because accreditation is almost exclusively concerned with process to the exclusion of product evaluation. He predicted that official doctoral program reviews within states that combined internal institutional review with inter-institutional reviews are the wave of the future.

In summary, institutional accreditation which includes graduate program evaluation appears to be acceptable to the higher education community. Specialized accreditation of graduate programs that grant the first professional degree also seems acceptable. Dressel (1978) identified seven general and twenty-four specific principles to be considered regarding review and accreditation of graduate programs. General principle #7 reads:

> Specialized accreditation should, in general, be avoided because it tends to support or confirm narrowness and conformity in the graduate student experiences and to retard the interaction and evaluation of graduate degree programs. (p. 34)

SPECIALIZED ACCREDITATION OF DOCTORAL PROGRAMS IN NURSING

The development of doctoral programs in nursing is a relatively recent phenomenon. Prior to 1960, only three universities offered doctoral degrees in nursing. During the next two decades, the number was increased by 17 bringing the total to 20 by 1980. Interest in doctoral education among nurses and within the higher education community grew in the 1980s. There are now 44 universities in the United States that offer nursing programs leading to the doctor of philosophy (N = 32); the doctor of nursing science (N = 13); and the doctor of education (N = 1). Two of these universities offer both the doctor of philosophy and the doctor of nursing science degrees, and one offers both the doctor of philosophy and the ND degrees. It is projected that five to ten additional programs will be established by 1990.

The rapid rise in the number of doctoral programs in nursing within the current decade has created some measure of concern within the academic nursing community. Issues of quality and accountability have been paramount topics for discussion at many meetings. Academic nurse educators are raising questions about the qualifications of nursing faculty, the adequacy of the research base, the availability of institutional resources, and the number of students needed for implementation of high quality doctoral programs in nursing.

In an attempt to address some of these issues, an invitational conference, "Doctoral Programs in Nursing: Consensus for Quality," cosponsored by the American Association of Colleges of Nursing and the Division of Nursing, Department of Health and Human Services (DHHS), was held August 1984. The complete proceedings of the conference were published in the *Journal of Professional Nursing,* March-April, 1985. One of the major outcomes of the conference was the development of "Indicators of Quality in Doctoral Programs in Nursing" which were sent to participating institutions for faculty review. The indicators were refined, assessed for comparability with the Holzemer Report (1986), and endorsed as a position statement of the American Asssociation of College of Nursing (AACN), in Fall 1986 as applicable to the doctor of philosophy degree in nursing (PhD), the doctor of nursing science (DNS), and the doctor of education in nursing (EdD). In approving the position statement, the membership of the AACN noted that *"the indicators are intended to be used to facilitate peer review of existing and proposed programs. They are not to be used as criteria for accreditation"* (Position Statement, 1987, p. 72). This conditional statement appended to the AACN Position Statement appeared to suggest that academic nurse executives were not supportive of specialized accreditation for doctoral programs in nursing.

In order to validate this perception, in June of 1987, I conducted a mail survey of deans, or their designees, who are administratively responsible for currently operational doctoral programs in nursing. The survey was simple in format, asking only whether the respondent *did* or *did not* support specialized accreditation of doctoral programs in nursing. The respondents also were asked to provide rationale for their opinion. The survey population was advised that information received would be used in this publication but that individual responses would be held in confidence. Academic nurse executives are apparently quite willing to publicly share their views on the issue because all but one of the responses were signed.

Twenty-four (54%) usable responses were returned. Nineteen of the 24 respondents (80%) indicated that they *did not* support specialized accreditation of doctoral programs in nursing; three (13%) supported specialized accreditation. The two (7%) remaining respondents did not select a specific option, choosing instead to provide rationale both pro and con.

Several general themes emerged among the respondents who replied in the negative. In essence, these respondents believed that existing mechanisms for the review and approval of doctoral programs such as regional institutional accreditation, cyclical internal reviews by the university graduate faculty and, where required, external review by the higher education state agency were adequate and appropriate. The view was strongly held that doctoral programs in nursing should meet the same standards as other disciplines within universities. Many respondents indicated that by meeting the standards established for other disciplines who had advanced further than nursing in their scholarly evolution, the development of excellence in nursing programs was promoted. Reference was frequently made to the AACN Position Statement, "Indicators of Quality in Doctoral Programs in Nursing," as a baseline tool for program development and evaluation.

In summary, the respondents were of the opinion that there is no additive value to specialized accreditation of doctoral programs in nursing. For several respondents, specialized accreditation was perceived as having the potential for limiting innovation, controlling curriculum and hence, creating conformity, reducing autonomy, and ultimately increasing expenditure of funds that might better be used to enhance program development. Whereas proliferation of doctoral programs in nursing and related issues of quality were of concern, the respondents were consistent in the opinions that these problems could best be controlled by existing review mechanisms.

The two respondents who provided rationale both in support of and in opposition to specialized accreditation of doctoral programs in nursing offered similar reasons as those described above for not supporting specialized accreditation. Reasons given in support of specialized accreditation focused primarily on "the need to limit the proliferation of programs."

The proliferation of doctoral programs in nursing and a concern for quality were the primary issues cited by the three respondents who supported specialized accreditation of doctoral programs in nursing. One respondent cited that "peer review" contributed to program quality. To assure peer review in specialized accreditation of doctoral programs in nursing, the respondent would require that both the visiting team and the review board be comprised of members responsible for administration and/or teaching in doctoral programs in nursing. In addressing the issue of quality, yet another respondent indicated that specialized accreditation could provide "identified standards for comparison across programs." Currently, accreditation is a voluntary process; thus, comparison across programs, if it were possible, would be limited to those programs acceding to the specialized accreditation process. Additionally, as noted elsewhere, accrediting agencies provide only a listing of accredited programs and this "listing" merely indicates that the majority, not all, of the stated criteria have been met. No comparative or evaluative data are made available to the public nor are programs accorded a rating score. It would thus seem that comparisons across programs would not be possible within the existing system.

CONCLUSION

Voluntary accreditation is a reality in higher education. Specialized accreditation is also a reality but its acceptance appears to be limited to programs leading to the first professional degree (there are some exceptions). Despite the general acceptance of both institutional and specialized education, criticism of the process and questions about the value and purpose of accreditation still abound.

In considering the question of specialized accreditation for doctoral programs in nursing one must ask if the presumed purposes of accreditation can best be achieved through this mechanism rather than any other mechanism. The goal of certifying to the public that an institution has met established standards is met by the regional association accreditation process. It is true that institutional accreditation does not examine any one program in depth as does the specialized accreditation process; however, the need for in-depth review of doctoral programs appears to be adequately addressed by evaluative mechanisms that take place under the auspices of the university graduate faculty.

Inasmuch as the federal government accepts the accreditation lists of the regional associations as one basis of eligibility for federal funds, specialized accreditation of doctoral programs in nursing is not a necessary qualifying condition.

Peer review is considered to be a constructive aspect of the accreditation review process. Specialized higher education accrediting agencies generally use faculty from a specific discipline or profession as reviewers. In contrast, regional accrediting agencies generally use as reviewers, faculty from many disciplines drawn from institutions with a Carnegie classification comparable to that of the institution being evaluated. Acknowledgement of a peer group is, of course, open to both subjective and objective interpretation. The majority of respondents to the survey previously reported clearly identified the peer group for doctoral programs in nursing as faculty from research-oriented doctoral programs regardless of discipline.

The goal of assisting students in deciding which institution to attend is as well met by institutional accreditation as by specialized accreditation, except perhaps in the case of programs leading to the first professional degree. Students pursuing advanced graduate study are more apt to choose an institution based on the recognized scholarly productivity of the faculty than on the type of accreditation the institution has been granted.

Whereas there is little or no empirical evidence to support the relationship between accreditation and quality in higher education, accountability of faculty must, for now, remain within the purview of the graduate faculty of each institution.

While it is conceded that accreditation is influential in the elimination of mediocrity in higher education, there is no evidence to indicate tha accreditation fosters the development of bastions of excellence.

One survey respondent succinctly summarized the issue of specialized accreditation for doctoral education in nursing by stating,

> . . . We do not yet fully know what nursing knowledge is and yet there is movement afoot to prescribe how it is to be gotten and from whom. Creative thinking cannot be prescribed. It's like trying to produce a great work of art by a "paint by numbers system" and that is precisely what specialized accreditation would have us do.

REFERENCES

Anderson, K. J. (1978). *Regional accreditation standards.* (Research Report Volume 2). Washington, DC: Council on Postsecondary Accreditation.

Astin, A. W. (1980, October). *Some new directions for accrediting.* Paper presented at the seminar on *Validation of accreditation standards* sponsored by the National Commission on Accrediting, Washington, DC.

Brubacher, J. S., & Rudy, W. (1976). *Higher education in transition.* (3rd ed.). New York: Harper & Row.

Caruthers, J. K. (1980). *Relating role and mission to program review. Postsecondary education program review.* Boulder, CO: Western Interstate Commission on Higher Education. (ERIC Document Reproduction Service No. ED 184 486)

Council of Graduate Schools in the United States, & Council on Postsecondary Accreditation. (1978). *Accreditation of graduate education: A joint policy statement.* Washington, DC: Council of Graduate Schools in the United States. (ERIC Document Reproduction Service No. ED 153 589)

Council on Postsecondary Accreditation. (1979). *The balance wheel for accreditation.* Washington, DC: Council on Postsecondary Accreditation.

Demaree, R. H., Jr. (1980). Accreditation: What does secondary school accreditation by a regional accrediting commission tell the college admissions officer? *National Association of College Admissions Counselors Journal, 25,* 36–39.

Dressel, P. (1978). *Problems and principles in the recognition or accreditation of graduate education.* (Report No. 4 of the Project to Develop Evaluative Criteria and Procedures for the Accreditation of Nontraditional Education). Washington, DC: Council on Postsecondary Education. (ERIC Document Reproduction Service No. ED 165 568)

Griffiths, D. C. (1978). Doctoral programs must pass a new test. *New York University Education Quarterly, 10* (1), 2–8.

Harcleroad, F. F. (1980). *Accreditation: History, process and problems.* (AAHE-ERIC/Higher Education Research Report No. 6). Washington, DC: American Association for Higher Education.

Harcleroad, F. F., & Dickey, F. G. (1975). *Educational auditing and voluntary institutional accrediting.* (AAHE-ERIC Higher Education Research Report No. 1). Washington, DC: American Association for Higher Education. (ERIC Document Reproduction Service No. ED 131 765)

Hart, S. (1984, March). *Accreditation: What it is — what it could be.* Paper presented at the semiannual meeting of the American Association of Colleges of Nursing, Washington, DC.

Holzemer, W. L. (1986). *Quality indicators of nursing doctoral programs: Final report.* San Francisco: University of California-San Francisco, School of Nursing.

Lawrence, J. K. & Green, K. C. (1980). *A question of quality: The higher education ratings game.* Washington, DC: American Association of Higher Education. (ERIC Document Reproduction Service No. ED 192 667)

Levin, N. J. (1981). The accreditation-eligibility link. *New York University Education Quarterly, 12* (2), 10–18.

Lewis, J. (1983). Accreditation: Is it really necessary? Unpublished manuscript, University of Cincinnati.

Manning, T. E. (1982). Accreditation procedures and actions of the Commission on Institutions of Higher Education. *North Central Association Quarterly, 56,* 63–128.

McCloskey, J. C. (1984). Nursing accreditation: To what end? In. J. C. McCloskey & H. Grace (Eds.). *Current issues in nursing* (pp. 359–372). Boston: Blackwell Scientific Publications.

Millard, R. M. (1979). Postsecondary education and 'the best interests of the people of the states'. *Journal of Higher Education, 50* (2), 121–131.

Millard, R. M. (1983). The accrediting association: Ensuring the quality of programs and institutions. *Change, 15* (4), 32–36.

National League for Nursing. (1964). *Accrediting chronology: Major developments leading to the present status of voluntary accreditation in higher education and collegiate nursing education*. New York: Author.

National League for Nursing. (1985). *Policies and procedures of accreditation for programs in nursing education* (5th ed.). New York: Author.

Newton, M. C. (1966). NLN accreditation: From four viewpoints. *Nursing Outlook, 14* (3), 48–51.

Petersen, D. G. (1978). Accrediting standards and guidelines: A profile. *Educational Record, 59* 305–313.

Position statement: Indicators of quality in doctoral programs in nursing. (1987). *Journal of Professional Nursing, 3,* 72–74.

Proceedings of doctoral programs in nursing: Consensus for quality. (1985). *Journal of Professional Nursing, 1,* 90–121.

Rienert, P. C. (1949). The purposes and values of accreditation. *American Journal of Nursing, 49,* 468–470.

Scott, R. A. (1981). *Program review's missing number: A consideration of quality and its assessment.* Indianapolis, IN. (ERIC Document Reproduction Service No. ED 200 108)

Semrow, J. J. (1982). A brief history and background of the accreditation process. *North Central Association Quarterly, 15,* (3), 383–395.

Semrow, J. J. (1977). *Institutional assessment and evaluation for accreditation.* (Topical paper No. 9). Tuscon, AZ: University of Arizona. (ERIC Document Reproduction Service No. ED 148 190)

Shannon, A. M. (1983). The NLN accreditation study: Its relation to the CBHDP accreditation process. In *Accreditation and the future of quality nursing education.* New York: National League for Nursing, Council of Baccalaureate and Higher Degree Programs.

Trivett, D. A. (1976). *Accreditation and institutional eligibility.* Washington, DC: American Association of Higher Education. (ERIC Document Reproduction Service No. ED 132 919)

Troutt, W. E. (1981). Relationship between regional accrediting standards and educational quality. In R. I. Miller (Ed.), *Institutional assessment for self-improvement.* (New Directions for Institutional Research No. 29). San Francisco: Jossey-Bass.

U. S. Department of Health, Education and Welfare (1980). *Nationally recognized agencies and associations.* Washington, DC: Office of Education.

Young, K. E., Chambers, C. M., Kells, H. R., & Associates (1983). *Understanding accreditation.* San Francisco: Jossey-Bass.

7 GRADUATE NURSING EDUCATION AND NLN ACCREDITATION: ALLIANCE FOR EXCELLENCE OR PROMOTER OF THE STATUS QUO?

Frieda M. Holt, EdD, RN

INTRODUCTION

Nurses are exceptional in their pursuit of excellence. The rigorous standards used in developing, implementing, and evaluating educational programs are no exception. The development of standards should provide freedom for creativity and growth within a structure that identifies excellence. Explicit criteria can give that direction for excellence, facilitate planning, and serve as a basis for evaluation. However, misuse of criteria and standard setting processes can restrict, control, stifle, and maintain the status quo. Have nurses been so rigorous, committed, thorough, and detailed in their search for excellence that accreditation is a negative rather than a positive factor in the quality of nursing education?

The first question that arises is probably why is there a need for accreditation at all? Why not let supply and demand provide the market monitor for educational programs and allow creative nontraditional programs to flourish "if their products will sell?" Products of poor quality would soon be revealed and schools producing those graduates would close. There would be freedom for individual institutions to develop their own programs to fit their own needs and they would control their own standards. The states could license them if necessary; or there could be institutional licensure. Such an approach would not be too different from the early stages of nurse training when hospital diploma schools were first initiated. Hopefully, both the public and the nursing discipline are aware of enough history to know that these free standing types of educational programs have no place in the modern era of the twenty-first century.

PURPOSE AND DEFINITION OF ACCREDITATION

Accreditation of educational programs in the United States is voluntary. It is the choice of the institution. It may well be that most institutions seek accreditation for prestige or financial gain. However, the act is also a philosophical statement by the institution—that it wishes to adhere to the standards that the discipline has defined, standards that protect the quality of education, public safety, and the profession itself against detrimental influences. Accreditation provides a mechanism for self-examination and self-improvement. It assures students of accountability in their education and preparation for future study. Accreditation ensures that each program receives periodic assessments, which point out shortcomings, acknowledge achievements, and provide stimulus for self-renewal.

The major purpose of accreditation in nursing education is to monitor its quality, (1) to provide standards for nursing education which ensure qualified graduates who can give safe nursing care, (2) to protect potential students by labeling programs which have the capability of providing sound education for nursing practice, and (3) to protect the profession of nursing by identifying the components of excellence and setting criteria by which to judge their achievement. The NLN's *Characteristics of Master's Education* (1987) and the *Criteria for the Evaluation of Baccalaureate and Higher Degree Programs in Nursing* (1983) contribute to establishing a common language throughout the discipline and should provide universally understood meanings to the labels of graduates.

The public is protected by three forms of credentialing mechanisms for health care workers. They include licensure, accreditation, and certification or registration (Flanagan, 1976, pp. 230–231). State licensure has evolved as a means of setting a minimum standard for those entering the health care system as practitioners. Professional certification is used to identify those who have attained specialized knowledge above and beyond that necessary to practice safely. Accreditation differs from both certification and licensure in that it recognizes the ability of an educational institution to impart a certain level of knowledge to students. As practiced within the United States, accreditation of an education institution does not necessarily encompass outcomes measures (i.e., measures of the graduate's capability). Thus, it does not directly reflect the student's ability to administer quality nursing care. Accreditation procedures do not currently focus on the quality of the outcomes; instead they assess the quality of the institutional components and processes (e.g., administrative, faculty, students, curricula, financial and facility resources, and teaching and evaluation systems) which are deemed essential in providing excellence in education. This is true of regional accreditation of universities as well as accreditation of professional programs of study.

Outcome Versus Process Criteria

In contrast, the classical European system of education focuses on evaluation of student outcomes as the means of defining excellence. The students ally themselves with mentors who supervise, guide, and direct individualized learning experiences which will prepare the students for a terminal examination for degree qualification. These experiences may include lectures, formal classes, informal seminars, readings, papers, laboratory courses, research, field work, and so forth. The emphasis is always on the achievement of the final goal and the means of learning/teaching are somewhat immaterial. The proof of accomplishment is within the student. The authority for determining that adequate learning has occurred resides in the examining body. The body of scholars responsible for the rite of passage (i.e., granting of degree) varies across institutions, disciplines, and countries in both qualifications and examining procedures. There is a universal deficiency in proven testing methodologies and measurement tools. The most prevalent means of testing is by written and oral examination by renowned scholars within the discipline. Needless to say, there are a number of potential weaknesses in the external examination system—the measurement tools, the brevity of contact, the potential differences in cultural practices and values, the dependence on the limited content within the final examinations, the use of thesis or dissertation research as sole indicators of competence, and the selection of one or two professors to represent world standards. Nevertheless, the prevalence of this practice in the academic world emphasizes the value placed upon the judgment of scholars, peers and professional colleagues in maintaining standards and high quality in educational programs.

In the United States specific remnants of the European system include the importance of the academic advisor and the research mentors, the preliminary and comprehensive examinations, and the writing and defense of the research theses and dissertations in graduate programs. Also retained in the American system is the importance of collective professional judgment as a valued and legitimate means to evaluate the quality of educational programs whether it involves the input, the process, or the outcome. Nursing has drawn heavily on this academic ideology in the development of the accreditation process.

Nursing educators are only beginning to examine the feasibility of including student outcome measures within the accreditation criteria. Outcome measures are used extensively throughout the teaching programs, but assessment of terminal outcomes for the graduates has not been a part of the accreditation process. Certainly, there is the need for more and better databased measurements of quality in nursing programs. Society has the right to greater accountability. However, it simply is not educationally sound or even possible to establish outcome criteria for accreditation unless there are valid, reliable, and economically and practically feasible ways of measuring the graduate's abilities. The Educational Outcomes Project (NLN, 1987, pp. v–x) was developed to identify, define, and apply outcome measurements to the accreditation process. The major foci of the study include (1) identifying what outcome measures are already being used by schools, (2) assessing how these measures of student outcomes could be improved, and (3) defining other methods which could be used to measure student outcomes. The study includes a survey of both accredited and nonaccredited programs (265 diploma, 787 associate degree, 401 baccalaureate degree, and 131 master's degree). Additionally, a content analysis is being carried out on 18 percent of all accreditation self-study reports from 1980 through 1986. At the completion of the study (planned for the end of 1987) recommendations will be made on if, why, and how outcome criteria need to be incorporated in the accreditation procedures. The study promises to be a major contribution in the identification and improvement of outcome criteria measures for data-based decision making in the accreditation process.

WHO HAS THE RIGHT TO JUDGE
THE QUALITY OF NURSING PROGRAMS?

One of the fundamental questions regarding any standard-setting/evaluation procedure is who has the right, the responsibility, and the capability of making a judgment. In the traditional academic world it is accepted practice that recognized scholars in the discipline provide the cognitive expertise, the prerequisite knowledge, and the responsibility for making judgments regarding the quality of work of professional colleagues. Professional disciplines have followed this academic model and, in fact, one measure of professionalism includes the ability of the discipline to develop its own knowledge base and monitor its own practitioners (Friedson, 1970, pp. 71–84). The wisdom provided by collective professional judgment is a valued means of decision making regarding standard setting and accreditation issues.

There is also concern that the lay public have opportunity to give input and have some say into decisions that affect their well-being. The balance between the amount of professional control versus the amount of public control is an ongoing debate in many fields that affect public welfare (e.g., education, medicine, and law). There is an overall public concern that the professionals may become self-serving and protect their own interests rather than make decisions that direct the discipline toward serving the needs of society. There is no doubt that an intricate balance exists. The tension between the short-term needs of the current market place as seen by the consumer and the long-term needs of society as seen by professionals is constant. At times the public wants immediate solutions without regard to the potential future consequences. The professionals can also be accused of dragging their feet in facilitating needed change for fear of losing control or going far afield from the discipline's traditions.

The NLN and its constituent councils are fortunate in having both professional and lay memberships to bring debate to controversial issues. The Executive Committee, the Accreditation Committee, the Board of Review and Appeals Panels all have non-nurse representatives. Thus the collective wisdom of these decision makers includes both lay and professional input.

Accreditation of nursing programs is less than 50 years old. The joint boards of the American Nurses' Association (ANA), National League for Nursing Education (NLNE), National Organization of Public Health Nurses (NOPHN), National Association of Colored Graduate Nurses (NACGN), Association of Collegiate Schools of Nursing (ACSN) and American Association of Industrial Nurses (AAIN) established the National Accrediting Service in 1949, and the first lists of accredited schools of nursing were published in October, 1949 (Flanagan, 1976, p. 624).

CHECKS AND BALANCES

Since 1952, the NLN has been responsible for developing and improving the standards of quality nursing education through accreditation (NLN, 1986). The League is officially recognized by the Council on Postsecondary Accreditation (COPA) and the U.S. Department of Education as the agency responsible for the accreditation of master's degree, baccalaureate degree, associate degree, diploma, and practical nursing programs. The master's degree program is accredited through the Council of Baccalaureate and Higher Degree Programs (CBHDP), which adopts and applies criteria specific to the graduate level. The accreditation criteria are based on the *Characteristics of Master's Education* (NLN, 1987), which are developed by the Accreditation Committee, whose members are appointed by the Executive Committee. Both the characteristics and the accreditation criteria are voted on by accredited agency members. The faculty and administration of accredited baccalaureate and master's degree programs and members at council meetings have many opportunities for input during the process of seeking consensus on changes. Accreditation policies and procedures are approved by the Executive Committee whose members are elected representatives by the total council membership. Site visits are conducted by collegial peers (i.e., faculty and administrators from accredited schools of nursing). Decisions regarding accreditation status are made by members of the Board of Review and, when appealed, by the Appeals Panel. The membership of both of these groups are elected. The accreditation policies and procedures are reviewed at least every five years by COPA, and the CBHDP is duly recognized as meeting all the requirements (and standards for excellence) and providing all of the safeguards for fairness.

WHY IS THERE A PROBLEM?

The checks and balances are all there. And, yet, the term accreditation still strikes dread and terror in the hearts of many nursing educators and administrators. In others there is the stimulus of challenge or the calming effect of reassurance and validation. What causes these disparities? Is it knowledge or understanding of the process? Is it an affective response to risking one's work to public scrutiny? Is it the history of a devastating personal experience? Is it horror stories from others' perceptions of real or hearsay events? Is it a reaction to an external authority; a response to perceived loss of control? Or is it that the system itself is faulty or so variable in implementation that it generates a multitude of responses?

If educational systems are conceptualized in their simplest form, there are three components: *inputs,* which lead to *processes,* which lead to *outputs.* Alterations in either the inputs or the processes affect the outcomes. The outcomes are also subject to question if the expectations were unclear, the measurement techniques were inadequate, the evaluators were poorly trained, or the interpretation of results was skewed to fit the philosophical bent of the individual interpreter.

Examination of the input, process, and outcomes of each of the six phases of the accreditation process can identify potential sore spots and the impact of historical changes can possibly provide some clues to varying perceptions. Perhaps then the question can be answered: Does accreditation of graduate programs facilitate excellence or promote the status quo?

ELIGIBILITY TO APPLY FOR NLN ACCREDITATION—PHASE I

The variations among institutions wanting accreditation for master's degree nursing programs is probably the greatest factor among the inputs of the eligibility phase. It is traditionally assumed that (1) graduate education takes place in a regionally accredited university that has multiple graduate programs in other disciplines, (2) the master's degree program builds on a body of knowledge developed within the discipline at the baccalaureate level, and (3) there is a planned program of study with identifiable faculty, students, courses, facilities, and so forth. However, in nursing education there are programs in single-purpose institutions which are not part of a university or college setting, there are programs that have no structured study requirements or course offerings which grant credits/degrees through testing, and the title of master's degree has been given to several types of programs.

Given that such a variety of institutions and programs have thus far met the accreditation eligibility requirements, there certainly can be no argument that the status quo is a problem at this phase. Indeed, there is widespread concern that the eligibility criteria are too broad to protect either the interests of the public or those of the discipline of nursing. The eligibility criteria are constructed to serve programs in all councils—could it be that accommodating to the needs of practical nursing and diploma degree programs has paved the way to the destruction of both the integrity and the universal understanding of degree titling of the programs in the traditional degree-granting academic setting? The opponents of open eligibility cite both ethical and legal concerns regarding the time, energy, and resources expended by any program seeking accreditation if the nature of the parent institution and/or nursing program does not meet the accreditation standards of the Council to which it is applying. The importance of the eligibility phase in the total accreditation process is frequently underestimated. It certainly is an area that could benefit from additional review and clarification by the NLN Accreditation Committee and Board of Directors.

APPLICATION FOR ACCREDITATION BY THE CBHDP—PHASE II

The administration and faculty of a nursing program should carefully consider whether the school is ready for initial application for accreditation. The program should be relatively stable in terms of university and school administration, faculty, students, curriculum, fiscal resources, and clinical agency support. The university administrators supply understanding and support to the site visitors; they must be able to articulate the interrelationships and role of the nursing program within the larger institution to help site visitors validate and interpret questions in the self-study report.

The nursing school's dean or director plays a key role in the accreditation process. The nursing administrator needs to know the history of issues, and at least identify with and be able to interpret the goals and objectives of the programs. The dean or director sets the stage with positive or negative expectations in the orientation of the university officials, faculty, students, and agency personnel for the accreditation process. The level of understanding and attitude toward accreditation expressed by the nursing leadership will permeate every phase of the process and influence every level of involvement. The dean or director's self-confidence, knowledge and perception of the process as a helpful mechanism can provide the reassurance needed by those experiencing accreditation for the first time.

A new curriculum should be fully implemented and an old one should be relatively stable. The self-study report is a written "snapshot" of an ongoing curriculum that is probably undergoing continual minor changes; however, major curriculum revisions should precede the self-study phase so faculty can study and present an ongoing curriculum rather than trying to create and evaluate a new one at the same time. The intent of an accreditation visit is to see a program in place and evaluate its implementation through the presentation by its faculty, students, and administrators.

Professional accreditation differs from university, state, and regional evaluation activities in that it focuses exclusively on the nursing program and its achievements. It is important to educate those involved in the professional accreditation process because it differs from other accreditation processes in purpose, focus, methodology, and decision making. If used well, the nursing program's self-study report and the site visit provide multiple opportunities to showcase the nursing programs. Professional accreditation is national in scope and provides validation of how the program measures up to national professional standards. It is "proof" from the outside world that the program, school, or university are performing up to or above national standards. As an outside influence, it can be used to provide education or an impetus for change—to the nursing faculty for needed evaluation and curriculum revision; to the university administrators for additional budget, space, or support services; to the graduate school, other campus disciplines, and clinical agency contacts for communicating activities and achievements in education, scholarship, and research. It is an opportunity to showcase and interpret the nursing program and the nursing discipline's current and potential contribution to health care and to society at large.

CONDUCTING SELF-EVALUATION AND PREPARING THE SELF-STUDY REPORT—PHASE III

Although self-evaluation is an ongoing process in any education setting, a major focused effort is usually initiated about 2–2½ years before an accreditation visit. The self-study phase is truly the most important and the most challenging for everyone involved including the institution, the CBHDP and the nursing program itself. For the institution it is the mechanism for self-examination and self-improvement. It requires current knowledge of the nursing discipline at the graduate level—this means knowledge of both general higher degree education and advanced nursing practice at the master's degree level to ensure that the nursing program meets the standards of both.

The self-study phase is challenging for the CBHDP is that its members must develop and keep current the *Characteristics of Master's Education* (NLN, 1987) and *The Criteria for the Evaluation of Baccalaureate and Higher Degree Programs in Nursing* (NLN, 1983), which provide the structure for the self-study. These documents are often the focal points of heated debate regarding the major issues in nursing education. At times, some of the criteria represent compromise among conflicting views. Use of neutral words that have standard meaning to all may results in general statements which can be interpreted in many ways. Even so, the *Characteristics of Master's Education* and the *Criteria* represent the best consensus possible of the collective thinking of nurse educators on the current norms and standards of excellence. The criteria will continue to require professional judgment in interpretation and use, but that is, after all, the nature of evaluation.

The challenge to the administrators and faculty of the nursing program is to conduct their self-study report using the accreditation criteria and then to write a report. The Self-Study Report is the presentation of evidence that a program meets the criteria. To administrators it is costly in dollars as well as in faculty time. To the faculty it represents hours of intensive labor, not only in writing but also in data collection and debate with colleagues on the content. To site visitors and board of review members it represents the major source of information about the program. If it is incomplete, disorganized, poorly written or too voluminous, their work is greatly increased.

The major efforts of the faculty should be to accurately portray the activities of the program, to provide evidence through data rather than opinion, to present the data as concisely as possible, and most of all to use the opportunity to objectively describe their accomplishments including both strengths and limitations. The self-study process should contribute to the excellence of nursing programs. The external stimulus for the program to undergo periodic systematic self-evaluation prevents the indefinite postponement of this type of comprehensive review. The successful outcome of the self-study should bring a sense of confidence and pride in the program's accomplishments as well as a sense of program renewal—the self-study report is but one small product of the potential outcomes of the phase.

THE ACCREDITATION SITE VISIT—PHASE IV

Every site visit involves intensive, hard work regardless of how good the program is, how expert and experienced the visitors are, or how well the visitors and school have organized and prepared. Still there are "good" and "bad" visits which potentially could affect an accreditation decision. Actually, most visits probably have some very positive and some less positive aspects resulting in mixed perceptions by various participants. The ability of the visiting team to project confidence and reassurance to the participants, to question and observe in a nonthreatening manner, and to interact as a professional peer rather than a judge enhances everyone's ability to have a "good" visit. Even problem areas can be examined and included in the report with tact and understanding. Observations and data need to speak to all the criteria, so reports must be comprehensive even if there is no new information and the observations just validate the Self-Study Report. From the perspective of many nurse scholars, there is too little time to observe as much as desired, to discuss individual observations adequately, and to write a report which can be edited and agreed upon by the whole team.

A recommendation that one hears repeatedly is to eliminate the Board of Review and have the final decision-making authority reside with the visiting team, as is done in regional university accreditations. This would require less detailed documentation by the visitors and provide the school with a decision at the time of the visit. A variation to this suggestion is that the visitors recommend accreditation status in their report to the Board of Review. Opponents to this position cite the inability of some visitors to address the negative findings in the open report even as it is currently handled. It is indeed difficult to stand in a public forum in front of an audience of administrators and faculty who have given their best to develop an educational program and tell them of the program's deficiencies, particularly if the deficiencies are serious and outnumber the strengths. Also, if a decision was made during the site visit, it would remove the opportunity for a program to submit corrections or make further explanations regarding observations or interpretations. Schools now have the opportunity to study the visitors report and to send corrections or additional information to the Board of Review. One of the checks and balances in the accreditation system is the variety of inputs and the amount of collective wisdom that enters into the final decision. The current role of the visitor, which is to clarify, verify, and amplify the self-study reports seems appropriate. They serve as the eyes and ears of the Board of Review. They are not the decision makers and hopefully will not set up false expectations either positively or negatively for the nursing program's upcoming accreditation decision.

Does the site visitor contribute to excellence or foster the status quo? That depends on the quality of the visitors, their skill in interacting with their colleagues as professional peers, and most of all their ability to gather data objectively and communicate their findings honestly. Their interaction with the school should be a positive experience for all participants.

EVALUATION BY THE BOARD OF REVIEW—PHASE V

Evaluation by the Board of Review is probably the most controversial phase of the accreditation process. It is at this stage that the evidence is weighed and the decision finally computed; thus, every aspect of the process is subject to criticism. The following discussion represents my observations and opinions as a participant in this phase.

In the late 1960s to the middle 1970s there was widespread consternation over the accreditation process and resulting decisions. It was an era when nursing education was in transition and the accreditation criteria mandated changes in some traditional patterns. In many institutions each specialty area had a separate curriculum based more on specialty content evolving from other disciplines than on shared concepts of advanced nursing practice. Curricula within a program varied greatly in the number of credits required for the degree, in emphasis on theory and research, in amounts of clinical experience required, and even in admission and graduation requirements. The introduction of a criterion to identify an explicit conceptual framework to provide rationale for curriculum content, course sequencing, teaching methodology, and evaluation strategies caused extensive revision of master's degree programs. Even programs in prestigious universities began to get major recommendations.

The concerns and needs of nontraditional study were gaining attention in the CBHDP. Nationwide there was a huge proliferation of programs which offered academic degrees to diploma graduates. Programs were developed for nurses but offered no additional nursing content. RN/BSN programs were also developing at smaller institutions. These programs would consist of a nurse director and two or three part-time nurse faculty for several hundred students. Frequently, such programs offered little upper division clinical nursing content and no supervised practice. Again, admission to master's degree programs was jeopardized.

The proliferation of "nursing" programs presenting serious quality control problems was not limited to the baccalaureate level. New master's programs had unqualified faculty, minimal numbers of students, multiple weaknesses in curricula, and virtually no financial support from the parent institution. Many were almost totally grant supported. As such programs were denied accreditation the uproar increased with accusations directed toward the CBHDP's rigidity and bias against innovation.

The CBHDP and NLN responded in various ways, reiterating support for innovation in nursing education. In February, 1976, the CBHDP published a position statement (approved by the NLN Board of Directors) supporting the concept of open curriculum in nursing education. In April 1977, a statement of concern was published regarding associate and baccalaureate degree programs for nurses that offered no major in nursing. In April, 1977 at the NLN Biennial Convention in Anaheim, California, two of seven program goals involved encouraging the development of innovative programs in nursing education and development of tests for nursing education that reflect new curricular approaches.

The membership still clamored for a major overhaul of the accreditation structure and process. At the 1980 CBHDP meeting in New York the central focus of the business meeting was change in the accreditation procedures. As a result of various resolutions, multiple changes were implemented by the Executive Committee: the members of the Board of Review and the Appeals Panels were elected by the membership rather than appointed by the Executive Committee; oral communication between the site visitors team chairperson and the Board of Review was again required during the presentation of each program as opposed to the Board having an option (this has since been changed back to optional contact); the dean/director of the nursing program was invited to be physically present throughout the complete presentation, deliberation, and vote by the Board of Review as opposed to being available by telephone for questions if needed; the time interval for reaccreditation was set at eight years rather than being individually determined by the Board of Review—the Board did retain authority for requiring interim progress reports and/or visits if indicated by deficiencies; on February 6, 1981 the NLN announced a major staff reorganization of its national office (the reorganization around functional lines gave structural independence to accreditation activities and established an accreditation division separate from consultation and continuing education services; communication to the membership about accreditation decisions was increased by sharing the numbers and types of decisions by both the Board of Review and the Appeals Panel).

These changes have been in place for a number of years and there appears to be greater satisfaction regarding accreditation within the Council membership. The criticisms now circulating focus on the interactions between the Board of Review and the dean/director, the group dynamics of the Board, the quality of deliberations within the Board before voting, and the potential for uneven decisions across programs. There is no doubt that the change in procedure required to accommodate the dean's presence throughout all deliberations on their school has affected the potential for free discussion and knowledgeable debate by the total Board.

A quick overview of the responsibilities of the Board members and the evaluation process may be helpful in understanding the issues. The number of programs to be reviewed have continued to increase and currently there are, at some times, as many as three full boards of 10 members each. Considerable preparation goes into each meeting of the Board of Review. To accomplish detailed program evaluation, the staff divides each Board of Review into three teams, with four on the team having the public member. Each team is balanced as well as possible to get a variety in specialty, type and size of institution, geographical distribution, and experience as a Board member. Most Board members have taught both baccalaureate and master's students, but obviously it is important in assigning schools with master's degree programs to have reviewers with extensive experience and expertise in evaluating graduate-level curricula. Each team is assigned several programs with one individual designated as primary reviewer for each school.

Each reviewer independently studies the program's Self-Study Report, visitors report, school catalogue and other materials seeking evidence for each criterion. Each of the three reviewers independently compiles a written report on each program identifying criteria which are fully met, partially met, and unmet. Areas for recommendations are cited and a tentative motion formulated. When the other two reviews are received, the primary reviewer combines all three reports into one and prepares a presentation for the full Board which covers all of the criteria and includes written recommendations in areas of agreed-upon deficits. Upon arrival at the League's national office, the team meets to review each program, reaches consensus on recommendations needed, and decides on a motion for accreditation status. This aspect of the accreditation procedures remained the same.

The Board Action

The changes in procedure involve how a program is handled when it reaches the total 10-member Board of Review. Prior to the changes, the programs were individually presented and discussed, recommendations agreed upon, needed revisions to recommendations identified, and a tentative vote taken. At the end of the week all program decisions with the edited recommendations were again reviewed, and a final vote taken. This double review is not realistic with the dean/director's presence throughout the review and vote. The previous procedure placed the first and final reviews on separate days, which would make it difficult for the dean. Also, the final discussion involved comparing decisions across programs and it would not be appropriate for anyone else to sit in on that discussion.

A second effect of the dean/director's presence is the potential loss of openness within the group to freely debate controversial opinions or issues related to the individual programs. Board members, like individuals everywhere, have occasional idiosyncrasies that interfere with objective analysis of particular issues. Previously, these inappropriate biases could be handled on the spot by open confrontation. Group process issues are more difficult to handle with an observer (i.e., the dean/director), who changes with each program and has a vested interest in the decision outcome.

A number of deans/directors have criticized the current evaluation procedure stating: (1) that the decision seemed final before the presentation and deliberation by the Board, (2) that the dean/director was not allowed sufficient input, (3) that the presentation was biased emphasizing some criteria over others, or (4) that they were treated with disrespect by the chairperson or other Board members. Other deans/directors have praised the process as opening up the "secret box" and demystifying the review process.

The Appeal Procedure

Programs receiving negative decisions have access to the appeal process and an additional review by the Appeals Panel. At one time the Appeals Panel could only reaffirm the decision of the Board of Review or recommend that the decision be reconsidered by the Board of Review. With the revamping of the accreditation processes in 1981, the Appeals Panel was given the authority to overturn the Board's decision and that has occurred several times. Although frequent reversals would be cause for serious questioning of the Board's decision making, the occasional reversal is probably an indicator of the proper functioning of the Appeals Board.

CONTINUING SELF-EVALUATION BY THE NURSING PROGRAM—PHASE VI

The decision of the Board of Review with its accompanying recommendations goes back to the nursing education program where the administrators and faculty may use the input for continued self-improvement. If the decision is negative, then the recommendations should identify the areas requiring change so that the program may qualify for accreditation. Likewise, recommendations with a positive decision identify areas needing improvement or change. All accreditation participants have struggled with ways of improving this feedback mechanism. Recommendations are intended to identify deficits and their seriousness without being prescriptive. They must be data based, related to specific criteria, and interpret the educational and nursing concerns in language that is easily understood by an audience that would rather not hear them. Improving the specificity of the recommendations is an area that requires continued attention because the recommendations are the communication link back to the school and serve as the Board of Review's input toward increasing excellence in all nursing education programs.

FUTURE DIRECTIONS FOR CONTINUED EXCELLENCE

The phases of the accreditation process have been explored for attributes which either encourage the status quo or contribute to excellence. There are nurse educators who believe the inputs and the process are not important in a system whose outcomes are positive. If the current accreditation process was merely maintaining the status quo, there would not only be stagnation in program development, but also accredited programs would look alike. In 1974 there were 65 accredited master's degree programs; in 1987 there are 145. Surely this is not maintaining the status quo.

Accredited master's degree programs have diverse characteristics. They admit (1) non-nurse college graduates for preparation as clinical nurse specialists, (2) associate degree and diploma nurse graduates for a fast track to multiple graduate nursing specialties, and (3) baccalaureate nursing graduates for advanced study in every conceivable nursing specialty. They prepare graduates for advanced nursing practice in functional role majors such as nursing administration, nursing education, and nursing health policy; in numerous clinical specialties; in dual clinical/functional role specialties; in generalist roles; and in a variety of primary care nurse practitioner roles. They are located on health science campuses, in large public and private universities, in small private and public colleges, and in at least one single-purpose institution. The variety in students admitted, the type of preparation they receive, and the different institutions in which they are housed indicate that the accreditation procedures do not encourage status quo behavior.

The level of cognitive and functional achievement inherent in baccalaureate and higher degree education is much more difficult to assess than the technical competencies at lower level programs. The complexity of the content, the scope of decision making, and the depth of judgment required for professional practice is difficult to measure. The master's degree graduate who is prepared for advanced nursing practice faces even greater challenges in the complexities of practice. The cognitive knowledge base can be easily tested, but the depth of judgment, and the advanced decision-making skills needed when the variables are in a constant state of flux require repeated observations and the best techniques in evaluation.

The current accreditation approach depends on assessing the traditional components of the educational institution for excellence. However, new innovative programs are eliminating various elements of these traditional components. How is the university setting assessed when the single-purpose programs sits alone? How are learning experiences evaluated when there are no programs of study in an external degree program? How are clinical competencies evaluated when there is no supervised clinical practice in the specialty areas? How do we educated the public and other health care professionals and employers regarding the differences among registered nurses prepared for licensure by a diploma program, an associate degree, a generic baccalaureate degree, a generic master's degree, or a generic doctoral degree? What do these innovations mean for accreditation? Are such programs simply not accredited because they truly meet only part of the criteria? Accreditation is, after all, voluntary. Students can attend nonaccredited programs and still take state licensure examinations. Can the problems be solved by redefining accreditation to focus entirely on outcome criteria? If it were redefined, how would it differ from individual licensure which tests for the minimal level of safe functioning? Do we continue to attempt to evaluate innovative programs with traditional program criteria allowing them to be accredited because they meet some criteria and can't be evaluated on other criteria because of the missing components? The next major focus for consideration in changing the accreditation process is the need to address better means of assessing nontraditional programs.

What criteria need to be looked at to evaluate programs whose creative nature omits the standard components of traditional educational programs in university settings? An institution seeks degree-granting status from the individual state's educational structure. If a single-purpose institution receives degree-granting status from the state, what is the responsibility of the professional accrediting agency in assessing attributes normally associated with an accredited university setting? Should there be additional criteria to ensure a learning environment comparable to that of an academic setting?

There is also a need for more detailed, acceptable evaluation measures for validation of nontraditional or prior learning. Diploma and associate degree graduates who wish to pursue further education must be assisted through baccalaureate education as quickly and efficiently as possible. However, the integrity and quality of professional baccalaureate education must not be compromised. Duplication of prior learning is frustrating for the learner and wasteful of economic and educational resources. Every means possible must be used to assess the level of the learner so that advanced placements can be made which allow for both degree achievement by the nurse and educational excellence for the institution.

If a program grants nursing degrees through testing, how should knowledge and safety in clinical practice be tested? Is it actually possible to assess a practice discipline through testing without extensive observation by professionals in a wide variety of clinical settings? How much and what type of teaching by faculty is essential? How much clinical practice is enough? How much can be simulated in the laboratory? How many clients must a student care for to gain enough experience to be competent? If testing the outcome is the only validation of learning, how much observation is needed during a test to establish clinical safety in the real world? What other types of learning experiences are required? Can they be simulated? If only testing is used, what criteria should be developed to assess the adequacy of the tests and the testing procedures?

There are those who would switch to a total outcome evaluation approach which would focus on a testing program for graduates and eliminate evaluation of educational components and processes. There is no argument from opponents that improved measures to test interval and terminal outcomes would enhance the accreditation process. During the forum for discussing accreditation criteria at the CBHDP meeting in Washington, D.C. in June, 1987 the membership expressed an eagerness to identify additional areas for student outcome measures which could be used to validate the educational process. There was, however, general reluctance to move quickly without adequate study of both the areas and measurement methodology. When the results of the Educational Outcomes Project (NLN, 1987) are available, current accreditation criteria should be strengthened to require evidence of outcomes measures in all feasible areas. However, the complexity of the competencies required for advanced nursing practice by master's degree graduates will no doubt preclude the shift to total dependence on outcome measures.

The world in which we operate as health professionals moves on rapidly. We need freedom to move with it. Health care is becoming more complex. All practitioners need greater competence. Nurses need more education—not just to be professional, but to be capable of understanding the complexity of health care knowledge and to be capable of delivering nursing care in the twenty-first century. We need a single voice in nursing—one that can compete and communicate with our professional and political colleagues. We need innovative educational programs, but within a well defined academic framework that is uniformly respected and understood by society and other disciplines within our professional health team. We need standards that provide the parameters for excellence and in so doing give real freedom for creativity and innovation.

We cannot assume that all nurses are equally qualified or equally competent to deliver nursing care. All registered nurses are not qualified to carry out the same activities regardless of state statutes. The associate degree and diploma graduates are not prepared to do what the baccalaureate graduates does and the baccalaureate graduate with experience is not as academically prepared to function as the master's degree graduate in advanced nursing practice. The nursing profession needs to increase the numbers of baccalaureate and master's degree graduates and all nursing education programs need to work toward this goal. If the nursing discipline could clearly define scope of practice and agree on titling for two levels of practice, then both the profession and the public would be well served.

SUMMARY

There is the need for a formal organization whose primary focus is nursing education: to monitor national trends in nursing, health care and education; to analyze critical issues; to provide a forum for national debate; to articulate a unified collective response; and to devise national strategies to address the issues. That organization must be responsible for collecting and deciphering information and providing the structure within which nurses, other members of the health care industry, and the public can work at improving the state of affairs in nursing education.

The NLN offers the combination of nurse administrators and educators with community members. This is the best combination for collective professional judgment available in nursing. The NLN provides a forum for debate among all nursing educators and concerned representatives of education, the health care industry, and the public at large. If the direction of nursing education is truly not good for the nursing discipline and for the public, the key actors are all available and hopefully the interest and welfare of the total society will prevail over the self-serving interests of a few. The current accreditation system for master's degree nursing programs is far from perfect, but in the final analysis, the bottom line must be this: who should decide what is and what is not good for graduate nursing education? Is it to be the public (by legislative mandate); is it to be nurse educators and administrators; is it to be all nurses regardless of their level of education, scope of practice, or visionary potential? The CBHDP makes full use of the leadership in nursing education with input from public members to define the characteristics, identify standards, develop criteria, and make collective professional judgments. The system is not perfect, but it represents the best collective wisdom available. Is it a promoter of the status quo? Certainly not to anyone who has witnessed the changes over the last 20 years. Even the continuing debates help to blaze the path to excellence!

REFERENCES

Flanagan, L. (1976). *One strong voice.* Kansas City: American Nurses' Association.

Friedson, E. (1970). *Profession of medicine: A study of the sociology of applied knowledge.* New York: Dodd, Mead.

National League for Nursing. (1983). *Criteria for the evaluation of baccalaureate and higher degree programs in nursing, 5th edition.* New York: Author.

National League for Nursing. (1986). Position statement on scope of NLN accreditation activities. *Nursing and Health Care. 5,* 235.

National League for Nursing. (1987). *Characteristics of master's education in nursing.* New York: Author.

National League for Nursing. (1987). *Educational outcomes: Assessment of quality—An annotated bibliography.* New York: Author.

8 EMERGING TRENDS IN NURSING RESEARCH: THE SHIFT FROM NURSES TO NURSING

Marylou Yam, MA, MEd, RN
Peri Rosenfeld, PhD

REVIEW OF THE LITERATURE

Since the 1950s, investigators have documented trends in nursing research (Simons & Henderson, 1964; Abdellah, 1970; Brown, Tanner, & Padrick, 1984).

In 1970, Abdellah studied the research projects supported by the United States Public Health Service Division of Nursing between 1955–1968. She reported that 22.2 percent of the studies pertained to health manpower, 15.6 percent to measurement of patient care systems, 15.0 percent to the nurse's role and its impact on the delivery of health services, 15.5 percent to faculty research grants, 11.4 percent to clinical research problems, and only 6 percent to model or theory development (p. 113).

In the 1960s nursing research began to shift its focus from studies on nurses and nursing education to clinical research. Brown, Tanner, and Padrick (1984) reviewed a sample of published research in 1952, 1960, 1970, and 1980. Their findings indicated that, in more recent years, there has been an increase in the investigation of clinical problems. For 1980, for example, they found that 63 percent of all investigations were in the area of clinical practice. They reported a significant decline in research on the nurse as well as a decline in research on nursing education.

During the 1980s nurse researchers set research priorities for the next decade. The 1981 ANA Commission on Nursing Research recommended that highest priority be given to research on the practice of nursing. Smith and Horns (1987) recommended that there be an increase in studies of cost-effectiveness and theory-based research (p. 24). Wood and Haber (1986) reported that a larger number of methodological investigations were needed (p. 13).

In addition, Simons and Henderson (1964) and Loomis (1985) analyzed nursing doctoral dissertations. In 1965 Henderson stated that "studies of the nurse outnumber studies of her practice ten to one and more than half of the doctoral dissertations were carried out in the field of education." Simons and Henderson (1964) reviewed 80 doctoral dissertations written between 1931 and 1955. They reported that 41 of the dissertations dealt with education, fifteen pertained to nursing care, and the remainder pertained to history, philosophy, and culture (pp. 124–125).

Loomis (1985) reviewed a sample of 319 doctoral dissertations between 1977–1982. She reported that 78.4 percent of the dissertations dealt with clinical research and 21.6 percent were related to such social issues as education, nurses, the economy, and politics (p. 115).

THE METHODOLOGY

With all of these studies as a frame of reference we obtained dissertation titles from deans and directors of 35 nursing doctoral programs in 1985 and 38 programs in 1986. This represents the entire population of nursing doctoral programs in the United States for those two years. A total of 170 dissertation titles were obtained from 1985, and 244 were obtained from 1986.

The Procedure

In order to analyze the dissertation titles, categories were developed to organize the dissertation titles according to the NLN's subject area headings. In 1985 the categories for the dissertation titles were clinical practice, nursing education, nurse characteristics, theoretical testing and development and methodological studies. The category clinical practice was subdivided into medical/surgical, maternal-child, geriatric, mental health, and community nursing. In 1986, the category headings were expanded to include nursing administration and historical studies and maternal-child was renamed OB/GYN, pediatrics, and women's health issues.

The clinical practice category included studies on client care, client assessment, diagnosing client needs, client conditions, and responses to illness. The nursing education category encompassed teaching methods, curriculum, evaluation tools, and roles and attitudes of students and faculty. The category on methodological research included studies on tool development to assess and diagnose client conditions on other measurement procedures, and on testing the reliability and validity of instruments. The nursing administration category included studies on job satisfaction/performance, staffing patterns, organizational structure, economics, and reimbursement. The category on theory development pertained to studies designed to test, apply, and explain theories related to the discipline of nursing. The nursing characteristics category pertained to studies on nursing roles, nurses' attitudes, and nurses' personality traits. Inter-rater agreement for classification was 100 percent of the dissertations for both 1985 and 1986.

RESULTS

Of the 170 dissertation titles from 1985, 117 or 69 percent were classified as clinical research. In 1986 the percentage dropped to 54 percent with 244 dissertation titles in the clinical research category. Although the percentage of research on clinical practice problems did decline between 1985 and 1986, this type of research still accounted for more than one-half of all dissertations. Within the clinical subcategories, medical/surgical nursing and maternal child nursing were studied most frequently in both 1985 and 1986. Geriatric investigations increased from ten in 1985 to twenty-two in 1986 while only one community nursing study was reported for the two-year period.

The second largest category for both years was nursing education. Dissertations on theory development increased from five in 1985 to fifteen in 1987 while the number in methodological investigations remained relatively constant over the two-year period with eight reported in 1985 and nine reported for 1986.

A few other trends in doctoral dissertation topics emerged from this review. For example, prior to 1986, women's health issues were so rarely researched that NLN placed all of these studies in the maternal-child nursing category. By 1986 there were sufficient studies in this area to warrant the establishment of a separate category for women's health issues. Historical nursing research dissertations were also a rare commodity until recently and a substantial increase in studies focusing on nursing service administration was noted; in 1986 this category represented 7.3 percent of the total studies reviewed.

CONCLUSION

It is apparent from the review that as the number of doctoral programs and students enrolled in them increased the quantity, quality, and relevance of nursing research improved substantially. The focus of doctoral dissertations in nursing has continued its shift from nurses to nursing and, in that process, the body of nursing knowledge has been enriched. In light of the number of doctoral nursing programs now operational or being planned, this trend will undoubtedly continue. Perhaps by the turn of the century the transition from research on nurses to research on nursing will be complete.

REFERENCES

Abdellah, F. G. (1970). Overview of nursing research 1955–1968, Part 1. *Nursing Research, 19* (1), 6–16.

Brown, J. S., Tanner, C. A., & Padrick, K. P. (1984). Nurses' search for scientific knowledge. *Nursing Research, 33,* 28.

LoBiondo-Wood, G., & Haber, J. (1986). *Nursing research: Critical appraisal and utilization.* St. Louis: C. V. Mosby.

Loomis, M. E. (1985). Emerging content in nursing—An analysis of dissertation abstracts and titles 1976–1982. *Nursing Research,* March/April, 113–117.

Simons, L. W., & Henderson, V. (1964). *Nursing research: A survey and assessment.* New York: Appleton-Century-Crofts.

Smith, M. C., & Horns, P. N. (1987). Forces guiding nursing research. *Nursing & Health Care, 8* (1), 23–25.